Multiple Choice Questions
In Clinical Radiology

MULTIPLE CHOICE QUESTIONS IN CLINICAL RADIOLOGY

For Medical Practitioners and Medical Students

Dr. Mohannad Salih Mahmud

Copyright © 2015 by Dr. Mohannad Salih Mahmud.

Library of Congress Control Number:		2015920501
ISBN:	Hardcover	978-1-5144-4381-1
	Softcover	978-1-5144-4380-4
	eBook	978-1-5144-4379-8

All rights reserved. No part of this book may be reproduced or transmitted in any form or by any means, electronic or mechanical, including photocopying, recording, or by any information storage and retrieval system, without permission in writing from the copyright owner.

Any people depicted in stock imagery provided by Thinkstock are models, and such images are being used for illustrative purposes only. Certain stock imagery © Thinkstock.

Print information available on the last page.

Rev. date: 01/15/2016

To order additional copies of this book, contact:
Xlibris
1-800-455-039
www.Xlibris.com.au
Orders@Xlibris.com.au

Foreword

Clinical Radiology is a rapidly developing and expanding specialty that requires an extensive knowledge and understanding of a wide range of specialties. The modern day radiologist has to be able review acute surgical cases whilst switching smoothly to trauma cases followed by oncology staging as well congenital anomalies. As a result the radiological examinations have reflected this requirement by testing the clinical and radiological knowledge of a wide variety of conditions.

This extensive book of multiple choice questions written by Dr Mahmud covers these wide spectrum of diseases. It is written in a format which is common in modern day exams and it's subject based separation of topics and questions makes it an ideal preparation book for the FRCR, part 2A exam which is in the same format. It is also very useful for other exams. The answers are widely researched and detailed explanations have been provided.

This book is not only an examination preparation book, however. It's detailed explanations allow it to be used from medical intern to experienced radiologist where it can be used to either acquire new information on a topic or as refresher. I am sure that this book of MCQ's with explanations will be very helpful to all in the medical field and I recommend it highly.

Dr Mohamed Ziyad Abubacker
MA (Cantab), MBBCh, MRCP, FRCR, CCST
Consultant Radiology,
King Faisal Specialist Hospital Jeddah
Jeddah
Saudi Arabia.

Preface

Radiology has become increasingly central to the diagnosis and management of all patients in current medical practice and having a good understanding of Radiology and its relevance to clinical practice is vital to medical practitioners from all fields and backgrounds, from medical student to senior consultants.

This book will address this need and will be of great value to medical practitioners at all levels.

The format is more of an exam based format, with 1000 questions and answers with each question having five statements with either true or false answers. Detailed explanations for each question have been provided which will enable the reader to assess his/her strengths and weaknesses and correct deficiencies in knowledge.

The topic parts of the questions are divided in six chapters.

Chapter I – Chest and Breast

Chapter II – Cardiovascular System

Chapter III – Genitourinary and Retroperitoneal System

Chapter IV – Gastrointestinal System

Chapter V – Neuro, skull, brain, and facial bones

Chapter VI – Musculoskeletal System

Those preparing for specialist Radiology exams will certainly find this text comprehensive and useful in their preparation, whilst even those from other specialties wishing to explore the radiological aspects of their syllabus in greater depth will benefit from these detailed question and answers.

Dr. Mohannad S. Mahmud
M.B.CHB, D.M.R.D London
F.R.C.R. London

1. Calcification of the pleura can occur in:
   a) Asbestosis.
   b) Coal miner's pneumoconiosis.
   c) Pleural fibroma.
   d) Old hemothorax.
   e) Cryptogenic fibrosing alveolitis.

2. The following may be associated:
   a) Pulmonary fibrosis and mesothelioma.
   b) Renal calcification and renal carcinoma.
   c) Pulmonary alveolar microlithiasis and renal calculi.
   d) Retroperitoneal fibrosis and methysergide therapy.
   e) Sarcoidosis and honeycomb lung in patient with diabetes insipidus.

3. The following are true in pneumothorax:
   a) It may be normal presence of little air in the pleural space.
   b) May be seen normally inpatient with tracheostomy.
   c) Spontaneous type of pneumothorax commonly seen in young males.
   d) Lung metastasis from pancreas, adrenal, or bones or Wilm's tumour can produce pneumothorax.
   e) Associated with active tuberculosis.

4. In bronchial atresia the following are true:
   a) Associated with pneumothorax.
   b) Usually traumatic.

c) Mucus commonly accumulates in dilated bronchi distal to the obstruction.
   d) Air trapping in the lobe or segment proximal to the obstruction.
   e) Obstructed distal lung can appear hyperluscent and hypervascular.

5. Septal lines (Kerley B lines) are seen:
   a) Infra cardiac T.A.P.V.D.
   b) Coal miners pneumoconiosis.
   c) Cryptogenic fibrosis.
   d) Due to dilated lymphatics.
   e) Sarcoidosis.

6. The following are true of scleroderma:
   a) Honeycombing lungs may occur.
   b) Alveolar cell carcinoma is a complication.
   c) Pleural effusions are common.
   d) Pericardial calcification is seen.
   e) Pneumothorax.

7. In alpha 1 antitrypsin deficiency:
   a) Upper lobe emphysema occurs.
   b) There is decreased flow to the low zones on a lung scan.
   c) Cor pulmonale develops rarely.
   d) Males are more affected than females.
   e) Associated with liver cirrhosis.

8. In cancer of the breast in the male:
   a) Left more than right.
   b) Carry the same prognosis in the female.
   c) Associated with the cancer of the bowel.
   d) Seen below the 25 years age.
   e) The mass usually diagnosed first when over 8 cm.

9. Following blunt trauma to the chest the following are true:
   a) The most common rib fractures are 4 to 9.
   b) Fractures of upper ribs should suggest underlying visceral trauma.
   c) Normal chest x-rays exclude ruptured diaphragm.
   d) Increasing hemothorax indicates continuing pulmonary haemorrhage.
   e) Pulmonary hematoma can occur without rib fracture.

10. In congenital lobar emphysema:
    a) Most common right lower lobe.
    b) Common in diabetic mothers.
    c) Cyanotic congenital heart disease is recognised complication.
    d) Diagnosed at the 2nd years of life.
    e) Can be multilobar, multifocal.

11. The following give expanding lesion in the rib:
    a) Eosinophilic granuloma.
    b) Hodgkin's.
    c) Tietze syndrome.
    d) Chondromyxoid fibroma.
    e) Myeloma.

12. In congenital cystic adenomatoid malformation:
    a) Bilateral symmetrical basal cystic lesion at birth.
    b) Associated with kyphoscoliosis.
    c) Respiratory distress at birth.
    d) Blood supply directly from the descending aorta.
    e) CT shows intrapulmonary mass containing multiple air-filled cysts, with probable mediastinal shift.

13. In bronchogenic carcinoma:
    a) Hyponatremia and raised urine osmolality.
    b) Gynecomastia.
    c) Acanthosis nigricans.
    d) Hypercalcemia without skeletal metastases.
    e) Thrombophlebitis.

14. Erosion of the lateral half of the clavicles is seen in:
    a) Hyperparathyroidism.
    b) Cleidocranial dysostosis.
    c) Progeria.
    d) Polyvinyl chloride poisoning.
    e) Klippel-Feil syndrome.

15. The following conditions give rise to pulmonary opacities and eosinophilia:
    a) Aspergillosis.
    b) Sarcoidosis.
    c) Tuberculosis.

d) Histiocytosis.
e) Polyarthritis nodosa.

16. In pericardial effusion:
    a) Normally less than 10 cc of fluid in the pericardial space.
    b) Cardiac tamponade required about 25 cc of fluid in the pericardial space.
    c) Commonly seen with pulmonary oedema.
    d) Hypertension is common.
    e) Pulsus paradoxus is present.

17. Immunosuppressive therapy can cause:
    a) Osteoporosis.
    b) Monilial esophagitis.
    c) Alveolar proteinosis.
    d) Pneumocytosis carinii.
    e) Reiter's disease.

18. In chilaiditis syndrome:
    a) Seen in about 0.25% of chest x-ray.
    b) May present with respiratory distress.
    c) Associated with renal failure.
    d) Common in young female.
    e) Associated with ascites.

19. In pulmonary hamartoma:
    a) A common benign neoplasm composed of cartilage connective tissue, muscle, fat, and bone.
    b) Endotracheal types presented with cough and/or haemoptysis.
    c) The vast majority located centrally.
    d) Can be calcified.
    e) Can cavitate.

20. In neonates the following are recognised features of the thymus:
    a) It is visible on the chest radiograph of over 40%.
    b) It is usually to both sides of the midline.
    c) Its size is constant in all phases of respiration.
    d) It causes an impression on the right margin of the barium-filled oesophagus.
    e) A fat line at its lateral margin may be seen.

21. A dyspnoeic child thought to have foreign body may have the following films:
    a) Inspiration chest.
    b) Expiration chest.
    c) Lateral neck.
    d) Laryngogram.
    e) A barium and cotton wool swallow.

22. Pectus excavation seen in:
    a) Down syndrome.
    b) Turner's syndrome.
    c) Marfan's syndrome.
    d) Osteopetrosis.
    e) Rickets.

23. Transient tachypnea of the newborn (wet lung) common in:
    a) Caesarean section.
    b) Prematurity.
    c) Maternal diabetes.
    d) Extensive amount of pleural effusion.
    e) Onset 24 hours after delivery.

24. The McKitty-Wilson syndrome may be associated with:
    a) Emphysema.
    b) Lung cysts.
    c) Renal agenesis.
    d) Pulmonary infarction.
    e) Paralytic ileus.

25. Short ribs seen in:
    a) Achondraplasia.
    b) Asphyxiating thoracic dystrophy.
    c) Paraplegia.
    d) Paget's disease.
    e) Hyperphosphatasia.

26. Pulmonary eosinophilic granuloma is:
    a) Characteristically a disease of female aged 40 years.
    b) Associated with miliary tuberculosis.
    c) A recognised cause of pneumothorax.

d) Associated with bone lesion in 15–20% of patients.
   e) Characterised by 1–10 mm nodules in the acute stage.

27. Chronic aspiration pneumonia in neonate seen in:
   a) Riley-day syndrome.
   b) Esophageal chalasia.
   c) Iron deficiency anaemia.
   d) Treatcher Collins syndrome.
   e) Macroglossia.

28. Honeycomb pattern CXR, soft tissue calcification, and bone changes can be due to:
   a) Fibrocystic disease of pancreas (mucoviscidosis).
   b) Tuberous sclerosis.
   c) Scleroderma.
   d) Hamman-rich disease.
   e) Old tuberculous bronchiectasis.

29. The following be true in Polyarthritis nodosa in children:
   a) Asthma.
   b) Radiologically stimulating rheumatoid arthritis.
   c) Generalised periosteal reaction.
   d) Microaneurysm of the kidneys.
   e) Cardiomegaly in about 14%.

30. In a child the combination of a lung lesion with mediastinal glandular enlargement suggests:
   a) Neurogenic tumour.
   b) Lymphoma.
   c) Tuberculosis
   d) Dermoid.
   e) Glandular fever.

31. In neonates hypoplasia of one lung may occur:
   a) With chest cage asymmetry.
   b) In associated with renal and gastrointestinal anomalies.
   c) In Fallot's tetralogy.
   d) In Potter's syndrome.
   e) In McLeod's syndrome.

32. In infancy an increase in the pulmonary vasculature is usually seen in the chest radiograph in:
    a) Truncus arteriosus.
    b) Total APVD.
    c) Fallot's tetralogy.
    d) Tricuspid atresia.
    e) ASD.

33. Egg shell calcifications seen on chest radiograph in:
    a) Sarcoidosis.
    b) Silicosis.
    c) Lymphangitis carcinomatosis.
    d) Pulmonary artery in chronic pulmonary hypertension.
    e) Adenomatoid malformation.

34. Retrocardiac lesion in a child may be due to:
    a) Collapse left lower lobe.
    b) Hiatal hernia.
    c) Thymoma.
    d) Para spinal abscess.
    e) Pulmonary sequestration.

35. Unilateral elevation of the diaphragm seen in:
    a) Normal.
    b) Scoliosis.
    c) Pregnancy.
    d) Ascites.
    e) Eventration.

36. Pneumothorax may be complication of:
    a) Secondary deposits from osteogenic sarcoma.
    b) Mesothelioma.
    c) Histiocytosis.
    d) Cystic fibrosis.
    e) Para-esophageal hernia.

37. Micronodular lung disease seen:
    a) Histoplasmosis.
    b) Histocytosis X.
    c) Melanoma metastasis.

d) Wegener granuloma.
e) Echinococcus.

38. Pneumomediastinum is a recognised complication of:
    a) Histiocytosis.
    b) Cystic fibrosis.
    c) Diabetic ketoacidosis.
    d) Hashimoto's thyroiditis.
    e) Situs inversus.

39. In sequestrated segment of lungs:
    a) Is often associated with diastematomyelia.
    b) Is usually in the postero-basal segment of the lung.
    c) May communicate with the bronchial tree.
    d) Is best demonstrated by arteriography.
    e) May cavitate.

40. Pulmonary arteriovenous fistula the following are true:
    a) 65% associated with Osler-Weber-Rendu syndrome.
    b) On CT scan the feeding pulmonary artery branch and draining pulmonary vein are dilated.
    c) Mostly centrally in location.
    d) MRI is the best diagnostic modality.
    e) Associated with cor pulmonale.

41. A 50-year-old man, heavy smoker, asymptomatic on routine chest radiograph, single lung nodule, was discovered:
    a) HRCT scan strongly suggested.
    b) Lung biopsy is strongly suggested.
    c) Speculated edge indicating malignant in 90%.
    d) Diameter exceeding 2 cm indicating malignant in 90%.
    e) Follow up in 6 months is recommended.

42. In chest lesions:
    a) Dermoids are more common in the mid-mediastinum.
    b) Bronchogenic cysts occur in the subcarinal region.
    c) Intralobar sequestration lung is the most usually seen in the right middle lobe.
    d) In Hodgkin's disease normally involved group of nodes are the broncho pulmonary ones.
    e) Ganglioneuromas occur in the posterior mediastinum.

43. Air bronchogram on chest radiograph seen:
    a) An infant.
    b) An area of Hodgkin's disease.
    c) A rheumatoid nodule.
    d) A metastasis from a renal cortical carcinoma.
    e) An alveolar cell carcinoma.

44. Cavitation of the lung occurs in:
    a) Rheumatoid arthritis.
    b) Infarcts.
    c) Closed chest trauma.
    d) Scleroderma.
    e) Wegener's syndrome.

45. The following are true:
    a) Proximal bronchial dilatation is a sign of Aspergillosis.
    b) In pulmonary artery stenosis the degree of post-stenotic dilatation indicates degree of stenosis.
    c) Subvalvar aortic stenosis is associated with infantile hypercalcemia.
    d) Pneumothorax may associate with endometriosis.
    e) Pneumothorax may associate with hypospadias.

46. The ribs are recognised sites of:
    a) Chondroblastoma.
    b) Osteoid osteoma.
    c) Osteochondroma.
    d) Fibrous dysplasia.
    e) Non-ossifying fibroma.

47. Bronchiectasis may be caused by:
    a) Pulmonary TB.
    b) Aspergillosis.
    c) Pulmonary hamertoma.
    d) Mucoviscidosis.
    e) Dextrocardia.

48. The following statements concern bird fanciers lung:
    a) The first radiological sign is a widespread pulmonary nodulation.
    b) Pleural effusions are common.

c) Repeated exposure of small amounts of antigen leads to shrinkage of upper lobes.
d) Large areas of consolidation may occur.
e) There is usually improvement following removal of antigen source.

49. There is definite association between asbestosis and:
a) Cancer of bronchus.
b) Cancer of larynx.
c) Mesothelioma.
d) Cancer of nasopharynx.
e) Cancer of kidney.

50. Calcification in the lungs can occur in:
a) Actinomycosis.
b) Coccidioidomycosis.
c) Histoplasmosis.
d) Toxoplasmosis.
e) Ornithosis.

51. Diffuse fine granular shadows occur in the lungs of neonates in:
a) Pneumocystic pneumonia.
b) Respiratory distress syndrome.
c) Meconium aspiration.
d) Cytomegalovirus pneumonia.
e) Transient tachypnea of the newborn.

52. Mediastinal emphysema occurs in:
a) Diabetes ketoacidosis.
b) Asthma.
c) Ruptured Meckel's diverticulum.
d) Pneumocytosis pneumonia.
e) Hiatus hernia.

53. The radiological appearance of narrow posterior ribs is seen in (so-called ribbon ribs):
a) Poliomyelitis.
b) Rheumatoid arthritis.
c) Pectus excavus.
d) Diastromatomyelia.
e) Thalassemia.

54. In Kartagener's syndrome:
    a) Always dextrocardia present.
    b) Abnormal sinuses.
    c) Normal lungs.
    d) Situs inversus.
    e) Pericardial effusion.

55. Lung changes may be seen following treatment with:
    a) Nitrofurantoin.
    b) Busulfan.
    c) Methylsergide.
    d) Pituitary sniff.
    e) Thymoxamine.

56. Pneumomedstinum is found in:
    a) Diabetic ketoacidosis.
    b) Marfan's syndrome.
    c) Intrathoracic endometriosis.
    d) Asthma.
    e) Traction diverticulum of the oesophagus.

57. Apparent elevation of a normally sited diaphragm in a chest x-ray may be due to:
    a) Mediastinal emphysema.
    b) Pulmonary infarction.
    c) Rupture of the diaphragm.
    d) Intrapulmonary effusion.
    e) Obesity.

58. Pleural effusion is common in:
    a) Histocytosis.
    b) Sarcoidosis.
    c) Cryptogenic fibrosis.
    d) T.B. in an adolescent.
    e) Heart failure.

59. The following cause pulmonary calcification:
    a) Hamertoma.
    b) Chickenpox pneumonia.
    c) Renal failure.

d) Histoplasmosis.
e) Alveolar cell carcinoma.

60. The following are true of Wagner's granulomatosis:
    a) Destruction of nasal septum.
    b) Pulmonary cavitation.
    c) Cardiac aneurysms.
    d) Renal failure.
    e) Die in respiratory failure.

61. CT diagnosis of calcification in lung nodule:
    a) Calcified nodule is commonly benign lesion.
    b) Calcification in lung tumours is typically punctuated or stripped and eccentric within the nodule.
    c) Soft tissue setting is best detecting calcium.
    d) Bone window setting is an ideal for detecting calcified nodule.
    e) More than 50% of carcinomas contain calcium.

62. The following may be seen in mucovisidsitosis (cystic fibrosis) on CT scan:
    a) Fingerlike mucus plugging associated with atelectasis.
    b) Periseptal emphysema.
    c) Emphysematous bullae.
    d) Bronchogenic cyst.
    e) Pleural effusion.

63. In miliary tuberculosis:
    a) Represents only about 2% of all active tuberculosis.
    b) Bronchogenic spread tends to produces pulmonary calcification.
    c) Risk of meningitis is high in children.
    d) Self-limiting disease is possible.
    e) Hepatosplenomegaly and/or lymphadenopathy are rare.

64. The statements are true in atelectasis of the left lower lobe:
    a) Is loss of volume of the left lower lobe due to bronchial obstruction.
    b) Elevation of the left hemidiaphragm with over aeration of the opposite lung.
    c) Posterior displacement of the major fissure on the lateral view.
    d) Silhouetting of all left hemidiaphragm may be present.
    e) Hilum remain in situ is a feature.

65. In hyaline membrane disease:
    a) Changes do not occur in under 24 hours.
    b) Diaphragms are low in position.
    c) Associated with prematurity.
    d) May show interstitial emphysema.
    e) Associated with irradiation during pregnancy.

66. In Atypical mycobacteremia:
    a) Usually results in fibrosis.
    b) Thin walled cavities are seen.
    c) Predominantly mid zone.
    d) Resistant to usual drugs.
    e) Pleural effusion is common.

67. In bronchopulmonary dysplasia:
    a) The lungs are overinflated.
    b) Asthma is recognised permanent complication.
    c) Pleural effusion is common.
    d) Conventional radiography is the study of choice.
    e) Constrictive pericarditis is recognised common association.

68. Feature of pulmonary alveolar proteinosis are:
    a) Cardiomegaly.
    b) Pulmonary edema.
    c) Pleural effusion.
    d) Sudden dyspnea with fever.
    e) Patching of ground-glass opacities bilaterally with interlobular interstitial thickening seen on CT scan.

69. In cavitary pulmonary metastases:
    a) Pulmonary lymphoma commonly cavitate.
    b) Primary lung carcinoma cavitate more frequently than metastatic lesion to the lung.
    c) Osteosarcoma when metastases to lung tend to be calcified and may be associated with pneumothorax and/or cavitation.
    d) Cavitation within the pulmonary metastases is usually peripheral in location.
    e) Cavitated pulmonary metastases can disappear after removal of the primary lesion.

70. In pulmonary interstitial emphysema:
    a) Typical transient.
    b) Pneumomediastinum is a complication.
    c) High altitude is recognised association.
    d) Present at birth.
    e) Associated with congenital lobar emphysema.

71. In neonatal pneumonia:
    a) Febrile is common clinical finding.
    b) Tachypnea is rare.
    c) Pleural effusion is common.
    d) Treated by oxygen alone.
    e) Impossible to differentiate from hyaline membrane disease by chest radiography.

72. The following are true in near drowning:
    a) Muller's manoeuvre is a cause.
    b) May be due to persistent laryngospasm with dry drowning (pressure edema).
    c) Metabolic acidosis occurs in all types of near drowning.
    d) Hypervolemia occurs in sea-water drowning.
    e) Central extensive fluffy areas of increased opacity on plain chest x-ray.

73. The following are true in Histoplasmosis:
    a) Spain in endemic area.
    b) Radiologically simulated tuberculosis.
    c) Central calcification (Target lesion) on plain chest x-ray is pathognomonic.
    d) Popcorn calcification on mediastinal lymph nodes > 10 mm.
    e) Acute Histoplasmosis is mostly asymptomatic.

74. The following are true in thickened breast skin:
    a) Anasarca.
    b) Ovarian cancer.
    c) Sjogreen syndrome.
    d) Sarcoidosis.
    e) Oesophageal carcinoma.

75. Calsifying lung metastasis likely seen in:
    a) Osteosarcoma.
    b) Thyroid tumour.
    c) Glioblastoma.
    d) Testicular tumour.
    e) Meningioma.

76. The following are true in legionella pneumonia:
    a) Toxic encephalopathy.
    b) Osteomyelitis.
    c) Bilateral patchy bronchopneumonia on chest x-ray.
    d) Diarrhoea is usually present.
    e) Patient usually distress respiratory failure.

77. Bronchogenic cyst the following are true:
    a) May cause lung collapse.
    b) May cause hyperinflation.
    c) Most common seen at the apices.
    d) Is premalignant.
    e) Associated with cyanotic congenital heart disease.

78. The following primary malignant tumours can be bilateral:
    a) Breast.
    b) Suprarenal gland.
    c) Ureters.
    d) Lungs.
    e) Testes.

79. In ground-glass opacity of the lungs on CT scan:
    a) Is specific in pneumonia.
    b) Seen in hypersensitivity pneumonitis.
    c) Bronchiolitis obliterans obstructing pneumonia is typically present.
    d) Typically has a patchy distribution.
    e) Areas of increased opacity obscure underlying pulmonary vessels in most of the cases.

80. Disseminated miliary nodular lesion seen in:
    a) Tuberculosis.
    b) Amyloid disease.
    c) Sequestration.

d) Polyarteritis and vacuities.
e) Alveolar cell carcinoma.

81. Disseminated interstitial (Recticular-Reticulonodular) infiltrates seen in:
    a) Hemosidrosis.
    b) Histocytosis.
    c) Haman-Rich syndrome.
    d) Hydrocarbon pneumonia.
    e) Hyaline membrane disease.

82. Disseminated alveolar infiltrates seen in:
    a) Giant cell pneumonia.
    b) Alveolar cell carcinoma.
    c) Scleroderma.
    d) Tuberous sclerosis.
    e) Oxygen toxicity.

83. Pulmonary fibrosis (honeycomb lung) seen in:
    a) Histocytosis X.
    b) Lipoid pneumonia.
    c) Alveolar cell carcinoma.
    d) Mucoviscidosis (cystic fibrosis).
    e) Dermatomyositis.

84. Solitary pulmonary nodule seen in:
    a) Bronchial adenoma.
    b) Hematoma.
    c) Hamertoma.
    d) Arteriovenous malformation.
    e) Hemochromatosis.

85. The following are true in Reactive Airways Disease:
    a) Usually transient.
    b) Atelectasis are due to mucus plugging.
    c) Associated with microlithiasis alveolitis.
    d) It can be due to viral encephalitis.
    e) Sinusitis should be always be excluded.

86. Mobile mass in a pulmonary cavity (meniscus sign) seen in:
    a) Hydated cyst.
    b) Wegener's granuloma.
    c) Mucoid impaction.
    d) Aspergillus fungus ball.
    e) Tuberculous cavernolith.

87. Bone metastases that are usually purely blastic:
    a) Bronchial carcinoid.
    b) Breast.
    c) Medulloblastoma.
    d) Bronchogenic carcinoma.
    e) Prostate.

88. In sarcoidosis:
    a) Caseating granulomas.
    b) Bilateral hilar adenopathy.
    c) Erythema nodosum.
    d) Hepatosplenomegaly.
    e) Granulomatous meningitis.

89. In mediastinal teratoma:
    a) Usually asymptomatic.
    b) Anterior upper mediastinum in location.
    c) Containing ectodermal elements with cartilage and fat.
    d) Mature type of teratomas had bad prognosis.
    e) Dermoid contain only epidermis.

90. Congenital lobar emphysema the following are true:
    a) More in female at birth.
    b) Associated with PDA.
    c) Mortality 80%.
    d) Commonly at the left base.
    e) Asymptomatic in 90%.

91. Increased skin thickness on mammography may occur in:
    a) Duct ectaisa.
    b) Fibro adenoma.
    c) Abscess.
    d) Traumatic fat necrosis.
    e) Paget's disease.

92. In Tree-in-bud sign:
    a) Indicating benign lesion.
    b) Seen best on lateral chest radiograph.
    c) Central in position on chest images.
    d) Seen in Eisenmenger situation.
    e) Can be seen in active pulmonary tuberculosis.

93. Accessory breast tissue (Polymastia):
    a) Commonly location is the chest wall.
    b) May be seen in the knee.
    c) Associated with urogenital defects.
    d) Associated with vertebral abnormalities.
    e) Always a benign condition.

94. A 35-year-old man undergoes a routine pre-operative PA chest x-ray. The reporting radiologist notes that the heart is shifted to the left. The left heart border is indistinct and there is a steep inferior slope of the anterior ribs bilaterally.
What are the possibilities?
    a) Rickety rosary.
    b) Cushing's syndrome.
    c) Marfan's syndrome.
    d) Swyer James syndrome.
    e) Chung Strauss syndrome.

95. Analysis of pleural fluid aspirate shows:
    a) High cholesterol content in rheumatoid disease.
    b) High glucose content in rheumatoid disease.
    c) Raised amylase content in pancreatitis.
    d) Chylomicrons in thoracic duct obstruction.
    e) A protein content of more than 3G/100 ml pulmonary infarction.

96. There is definite association between asbestosis and:
    a) Ca. bronchus.
    b) Ca. larynx.
    c) Mesothelioma.
    d) Ca. Nasopharynx.
    e) Ca. kidney.

97. In nipple discharge:
   a) Commonly associated with endocrine.
   b) The first examination that will be performed in patient with nipple discharge is galactography.
   c) Sonography is typically used in this case.
   d) There is no role of MRI in nipple discharge.
   e) Galactography is not indicated unless the nipple discharge is spontaneous, unilateral, and expressed from a single pore.

98. On ultrasound of the breast, characteristics of benign mass are:
   a) Ellipsoid.
   b) Thin echogenic pseudo capsule.
   c) Hyper echogenicity.
   d) Gentle bi- or tri-lobulation.
   e) Speculation.

99. In gynecomastia:
   a) Hypogonadism.
   b) Cimetidine therapy.
   c) In the neonates and adolescents generally needs hormone therapy.
   d) Hormonal causes may be required mastectomy.
   e) May be associated with spironolactous therapy.

100. In breast implant rupture:
   a) Mostly intracapsular.
   b) Is best seen in on MRI.
   c) Change in the implant contour indicate extracapsular rupture.
   d) Detection of silicone implant ruptures is easily diagnosed on mammography.
   e) Ultrasound may demonstrate a snow storm appearance of an extra-capsular rupture.

101. In breast carcinoma:
   a) Infiltrating ductal carcinoma is the most common form.
   b) Dense irregular mass with speculating margins is a feature on mammography.
   c) Pleomorphic malignant calcifications are rarely present on mammography.
   d) Bilateral breast involvement is usually symmetrical.
   e) Axillary lymph gland involvement is always present.

102. In breast fibro-adenoma:
    a) Called breast mouse.
    b) A thin 'halo' is often seen around the lesion on mammography.
    c) Mobile, solid hypo echoic mass with macro lobulated, well-defined margin on ultrasound.
    d) Dense irregular mass with speculating margins on mammogram.
    e) Homogeneous enhancement with dark internal septae following gadolinium.

103. In breast cyst:
    a) Symptomatic palpable lump usually.
    b) The most common benign lesions identified in the breast.
    c) Caused by terminal ductal obstruction, dilatation, and fluid retention.
    d) On ultrasound well-circumscribed anechoic lesions with thin back wall and good through transmission.
    e) Hyperintense on T2W scans hypointense on T1W scans.

104. In flail chest:
    a) Pain on inspiration.
    b) Rib fractures always present.
    c) Airspace disease representing haemorrhage into the alveoli.
    d) Hemothorax is rare.
    e) Pneumothorax is rare.

105. Rat-tail sign seen in:
    a) Achalasia.
    b) Hydroureters.
    c) Bronchiactasis.
    d) Bronchus carcinoma.
    e) Billary duct carcinoma.

106. Exudates pleural effusion seen in:
    a) Nephrotic syndrome.
    b) Mitral stenosis.
    c) Tuberculosis.
    d) Complication of myocardial infarction.
    e) Penetrating injury.

107. Chylothorax commonly seen in:
    a) Tuberculosis.
    b) Fungal lung infections.
    c) Thoracic duct obstruction.
    d) Amyloidosis.
    e) Lymphoma.

108. Transudate pleural effusion seen in:
    a) Meig's syndrome.
    b) Ovarian hyper stimulation.
    c) Pneumonia.
    d) Dressler's syndrome.
    e) Hypothyroidism.

109. In thymus gland:
    a) More prominent on inspiration film.
    b) Sail sign appearance of the thymus gland on both sides of the mediastinum is normally seen on plain radiograph.
    c) About 20% of patient with myasthenia gravis have a thymic tumour.
    d) During infective illnesses the thymus often becomes smaller.
    e) Enlarged significantly in Di George syndrome.

110. Increased skin thickness on mammography may occur in:
    a) Duct ectasia.
    b) Fibro adenoma.
    c) Abscess.
    d) Traumatic fat necrosis.
    e) Paget's disease.

111. The following signs are related to the following condition:
    a) Water bottle sign and pericardial effusion.
    b) White pyramid sign and multiple myeloma.
    c) Coffee bean sign (bent inner tube sign) and sigmoid volvulus.
    d) Pancake vertebra (vertebra-plans) and eosinophilic granuloma.
    e) Cottage loaf sign and diaphragmatic rupture.

112. In irradiation:
    a) Changes occur only after 8 weeks.
    b) Constrictive pericarditis only occurs after 2 years.
    c) Pleural effusions commonly occur.

d) B-septal lines may occur.
e) Nephritis is common.

113. Air bronchogram rarely seen on plain radiograph in:
    a) An infarct.
    b) Hodgkin's disease.
    c) Rheumatoid nodule.
    d) Metastasis from a renal cortical ca.
    e) Alveolar cell ca.

114. Recurrent fleeting infiltrates on chest radiograph are caused by:
    a) Tropical pulmonary eosinophilia.
    b) Sarcoidosis.
    c) Infective endocarditis.
    d) Bronchogenic granulomatosis.
    e) Aspergillosis.

115. Causes of broncholithiasis:
    a) Histoplasmosis.
    b) Hyperparathyroidism.
    c) Sarcoidosis.
    d) Actinomycosis.
    e) Tuberculosis.

116. In pneumatocele:
    a) Usually multiple.
    b) Seen in all age groups.
    c) May contain air/fluid levels.
    d) May disappear without treatment.
    e) The majority occur as result of staphylococcus aureus pneumonia.

117. In mongolism (Down syndrome):
    a) Eleven pairs of ribs.
    b) Hypertelorism.
    c) Hypoplasia of the nasal bone.
    d) Iliac index is over 90.
    e) Hypoplasia of the thumb.

118. A 50-year-old man chest radiograph shows complete white-out of hemothorax and the trachea pulled toward the opacified side. The likely diagnosis:
   a) Extensive pleural effusion.
   b) Pulmonary agenesis.
   c) Pulmonary edema/ARDS.
   d) Total lung collapse.
   e) Diaphragmatic hernia.

119. In pulmonary contusion:
   a) Children are more susceptible than adult.
   b) It usually occurs secondary to penetrating trauma.
   c) Usually give a permanent lung damage.
   d) On CT scan typically seen as focal, non-segmental crescentic area of parenchymal opacification.
   e) Pleural effusion is a feature.

120. In hila region:
   a) The left pulmonary artery arches over the left lower lobe bronchus.
   b) The posterior aspect of the right main bronchus is seen as a thin stripe.
   c) There is a small bit of lung between the left lower lobe artery and descending aorta.
   d) The left pulmonary artery lies postero lateral to the left lower lobe bronchus.
   e) No normal structure posterior to the right upper lobe bronchus and bronchus intermedius.

121. HRCT anatomy of lung the following are true:
   a) The artery supplying the lobule reaches the pleural border.
   b) The smallest functional unit of lung is the alveolus.
   c) Secondary pulmonary lobules are best seen in the periphery of the lungs.
   d) The central broncho vascular bundle consisting of bronchiole and artery is seen 1 cm away from the pleural border.
   e) Secondary pulmonary lobule can have 10 acini.

122. In bronchiectasis:
    a) Classical clinical triad, chronic cough, excess sputum production, and repeated infection.
    b) Three major causes are obstruction, infection, traction.
    c) Pulmonary fibrosis and honeycombing lungs is best seen by high resolution CT.
    d) Associated with miliary tuberculosis.
    e) Associated with Kartagener's syndrome.

1.   a. True   b. True   c. True   d. True   e. False

Pleural calcification seen in organised empyema, pleural effusion, and hemothorax. Also seen in pneumoconiosis particularly tin, barium, asbestosis, and silicates. Old tuberculosis, histoplasmosis, and tongue worm (Armilliter) infestation.

2.   a. True   b. True   c. False   d. True   e. True

Pulmonary fibrosis can be associated with mesothelioma in several condition, e.g., asbestosis. Calcification occurs in 6% of renal carcinoma, may take the form of irregular areas scattered throughout the tumour.

Alveolar microlithiasis
- Very rare of unknown etiology characterised by myriad of calcospherities (tiny calculi) with alveoli.
- 50% familiar (siblings).
- Usually asymptomatic 70%.
- Dyspnea, cyanosis, clubbing fingers.
- Normal serum calcium + phosphorus levels.
- Cor pulmonale however may be a terminal sequel.
- Is not associated with renal stone.

Retroperitoneal fibrosis, unknown etiology, is proliferation of fibrous tissue in the retroperitoneal space. May followed the use of methysergide and other ergo + derivatives. The fibrosis may spread up to mediastinum and crura of the diaphragm.

3. a. False   b. False   c. True   d. True   e. True

Pneumothorax
- Present of air in the pleural space.
- Acute onset of cough, dyspnea, pleuritic pain, back or shoulder pain.
- Commonly 20–40 years, male: female – 8:1.
- Especially in patients who are tall, thin, fare, smokers.
- Catamenial pneumothorax is a recurrent spontaneous pneumothorax that occurs during menstruation and is associated with endometriosis of the diaphragm.
- Pneumothorax may be open, closed, tension. It may be sub pulmonic pneumothorax.

4. a. False   b. False   c. True   d. False   e. True

5. a. False   b. True   c. True   d. True   e. True

Septal Line (Kerley B Lines) are seen when the interlobular septa in the pulmonary interstitium become prominent. May be because of the lymphatic engorgement or oedema of the connective tissue of the interlobular septa. They usually occur when pulmonary capillary wedge pressure reach 20-25 mmHg. They are about 2-5 cm long and < 1 mm thickness, at peripheries of the lung best at the bases laterally perpendicular to and extended out to the pleural surface. Seen also in mitral valve disease, lymphatic metastases, thoracic duct obstruction, pneumoconiosis, Hamman-Rich syndrome, Sarcoidosis, lipoid pneumonia, radatio fibrosis and others.

6. a. True   b. True   c. False   d. True   e. True

Scleroderma (Diffuse Systemic Sclerosis) – Reynauld's ischemia of hands and feet may precede the typical atrophy and hardening of the skin and subcutaneous tissue. Gastro-intestinal and respiratory tracts may be involved. Honeycomb lung, fibrosis, and spontaneous pneumothorax may occur. Rare complication is carcinoma of bronchus, adenocarcinoma, or alveolar cell carcinoma. Pericarditis and pericardial calcification may also present.

7. a. False   b. True   c. False   d. True   e. True

Alpha-1-antitrypsine deficiency is inherited recessive disorder among Caucasians that may causes lung (emphysema) and/or liver diseases (cirrhosis). Smoking is increase the risk. Bilateral lower lobe emphysema present and upper lobe vein diversion. Commonly affected the males.

8.   a. True   b. True   c. True   d. False   e. True

The normal male breast is predominantly composed of fat that has no lobules and only rudimentary ducts. Therefore male breasts do not develop fibroadenomas. Gynecomastia occurs mostly in adolescent boys and men more than 50 years. Male breast cancer is rare about 0.2% of male malignancies mean age 70 years. Mammographic finding in male cancer are similar to those in female cancer.

Predisposing factors are:
1. Prior breast radiation
2. Klinefelter's syndrome

9.   a. True   b. False   c. False   d. True   e. True

Trauma to the Chest
The thoracic cage and its contents may be damaged by penetrating or non-penetrating injuries. The non-penetrating may be caused by blows, falls on the chest, blast injuries, and increasingly by car accidents, particularly of steering-wheel type.

Penetrating injuries are far less frequent except in times of war, usually caused by knife, glass sharpener, or bullet wounds.

Fractured ribs are common may be a faint hair-line or the dangerous flail segment. Flail segment is sucked in during the underlying lung. Pneumothorax and/or surgical emphysema of the chest wall at mediastinum and costal cartilage injuries are associated with blunt chest, as well as injured diaphragm, contusion, or laceration of the lung. Haemothorax may complicate open or closed chest trauma. Fat embolism is unusual complication of multiple rib fracture as well as laceration and rupture of a major air passage.

The heart, aorta, pulmonary arteries and veins, systemic veins may be contused or ruptured. Haemopericardium may be seen on result of ruptures heart or aorta, traumatic aortic aneurysm, dissecting aneurysm or mediastinal haematoma may result. Traumatic damage to the thoracic ducts may result in chylothorax and chylous ascites.

10. a. False   b. False   c. False   d. False   e. True

Congenital lobar emphysema is idiopathic, congenital progressive over distention of a pulmonary lobe. Classical imaging appearance hyperlucent hyperexpanded lobe, presentation with respiratory distress during neonatal period.

The predilection lobar is left upper lobe 43%, right middle lobe 32%, right upper lobe 20%.

The CT finding lucency caused by air distended alveoli, hyper lucent lung, the vessel attenuated and smaller than those in adjacent in periphery of lucencies not centrally located.

11. a. True   b. True   c. False   d. True   e. True

Expanding of the Ribs (Wide Ribs)
Localised or generalised – the localised wide rib usually seen in post trauma or infection tumour benign or malignant primary or secondary.

Some causes of wide ribs – Paget' disease, basal cell nerves syndrome (Gorlin). Infantile cortical hypertosis (Caffey's disease), rickets, hyperphophatasia. Also in Schmidt and Pyle's disease, fibrous dysplasia, and anaemia in general.

Tietze syndrome is a benign inflammation of one or more of the costal cartilage.

12. a. False   b. False   c. True   d. False   e. True

Congenital cystic adenomatoid malformation is a congenital lung mass of adenomatoid proliferation. Classically appearance, multicystic mass with air in cyst, present with respiratory distress, infection, or may be detected at prenatal ultrasound. There are three types depend on size of cysts at imaging and pathology, it may contain air. There is no lobar predilection.

Should be differentiated from sequestration, congenital diaphragmatic hernia, cavitated pneumonic consolidation.

13. a. True   b. True   c. False   d. True   e. True

Bronchogenic carcinoma is the most common malignant tumour in men. Men are affected more frequently than females. The incidence is greatly increase in heavy smokers and in urban than in rural community. Rarely accompanied with gynecomastia.
Type:
    1.   Adenocarcinoma 50%.
    2.   Squamous cell carcinoma (epidermoid carcinoma) 30–35%.
    3.   Small cell undifferentiated carcinoma 15%.
    4.   Undifferentiated large cell carcinoma < 5%.

14. a. True   b. True   c. True   d. False   e. False

Short clavicle are seen in many condition, congenital and acquired. The congenital includes progeria, cleidocranial dysostosis, and pyknodysostosis. The acquired is traumatic, inflammatory, collagen disease, e.g., rheumatoid or hormonal, e.g., hyperparathyroidism.

15. a. True   b. True   c. True   d. False   e. True

Pulmonary Disease with Eosinophilia
Eosinophilia is abnormally increased eosinophils in the blood. Also called eosinophilic leukocytosis several pulmonary diseases are associated.
    1.   Aspergillus sensitivity.
    2.   Asthma.
    3.   Drug sensitivity (e.g., Furadantin, penicillin, isoniazid, sulfa).
    4.   Eosinophilic leukaemia.
    5.   Idiopathic, acute (Lofter's syndrome).
    6.   Idiopathic, chronic (PIE).
    7.   Parasitic disease, including tropical eosinophilia.
    8.   Brucellosis.
    9.   Carcinoma (e.g., lung).
    10.   Coccidioidemycosis.
    11.   Desquamative interstitial pneumonitis (DIP).
    12.   Polyarteritis nodosa.
    13.   Wegener's granuloma.

16. a. False   b. False   c. False   d. False   e. True

Pericardial Effusion

- Abnormal amount of fluid in the pericardial space, defined as the presence between the visceral and parietal layers of the pericardium.
- Normally contains about 20–50 cc of fluid.
- Normal thickness of pericardium (parietal pericardium and fluid space) is 2–4 mm.
- Small effusions frequently produce no symptoms.
- Chest pain or discomfort with a characteristic of being relieved by sitting up or leaning forward and worsened in the supine position.
- Syncope.
- Palpitations.
- Shortness of breath, tachypnea.

Imaging Findings
1. Conventional radiography
   - Suggestive but not usually diagnostic.
   - 'Water bottle configuration' is symmetrically enlarged cardiac silhouette.
   - Loss of retrosternal clear space.
   - 'Fat-pad sign.'
   - Produced by separation of retrosternal from epicardial fat line > 2 mm.
   - Rapidly enlarging cardiac silhouette with normal pulmonary vascularity.
2. Echocardiogram
   - Study of choice.
   - Echo-free fluid between the visceral and parietal pericardium.
3. CT
   - May detect small effusions (50 cc).
   - Fluid-filled space surrounding the myocardium.
   - Early effusions accumulate posteriorly first.

17. a. True   b. True   c. True   d. True   e. False

18. a. True   b. True   c. False   d. False   e. False

19. a. True   b. True   c. False   d. True   e. False

20. a. False   b. True   c. False   d. False   e. False

21. a. True   b. True   c. True   d. False   e. True

22.	a. True	b. True	c. True	d. False	e. True
23.	a. True	b. True	c. True	d. False	e. True
24.	a. True	b. True	c. False	d. False	e. False
25.	a. True	b. True	c. False	d. False	e. False
26.	a. False	b. True	c. True	d. True	e. True
27.	a. True	b. True	c. False	d. True	e. False
28.	a. True	b. True	c. True	d. False	e. False
29.	a. True	b. False	c. False	d. True	e. True
30.	a. True	b. True	c. True	d. False	e. True
31.	a. False	b. True	c. True	d. False	e. False
32.	a. True	b. True	c. False	d. True	e. False
33.	a. True	b. True	c. False	d. True	e. False
34.	a. True	b. True	c. False	d. True	e. True
35.	a. True	b. True	c. False	d. False	e. True
36.	a. True	b. False	c. True	d. True	e. True
37.	a. True	b. True	c. True	d. False	e. False
38.	a. True	b. True	c. True	d. False	e. False
39.	a. False	b. True	c. True	d. True	e. True
40.	a. True	b. True	c. False	d. False	e. False
41.	a. True	b. False	c. True	d. True	e. False
42.	a. False	b. True	c. False	d. False	e. True

43. a. False   b. True   c. False   d. True   e. True

44. a. True   b. True   c. True   d. False   e. True

45. a. True   b. False   c. True   d. True   e. True

46. a. True   b. True   c. True   d. True   e. False

47. a. True   b. True   c. False   d. True   e. True

Broncheictasis may be associated with abnormal dilatation of the bronchial tree. The most common cause is post-infection, e.g., tuberculosis, Aspergillosis, Histoplasmosis, etc.

Congenital causes such as cystic fibrosis, ciliary dysfunction syndrome, e.g., Kartagener's syndrome, which is associated with dextrocardia. Macroscopic morphology subtypes are:
1. Cylindrical have parallel wall (tram track sign and signet ring sign).
2. Varicose Broncheictasis beaded appearances.
3. Cystic type is a severe from that can extend to the pleural surface and air level is commonly present.

It can occur also in late complication of inhalation of gastric contents (Mendelson's syndrome).

48. a. True   b. False   c. True   d. True   e. True

49. a. True   b. True   c. True   d. True   e. False

50. a. True   b. True   c. True   d. False   e. False

51. a. True   b. True   c. True   d. False   e. False

52. a. True   b. True   c. False   d. True   e. True

53. a. True   b. False   c. True   d. False   e. False

54. a. True   b. True   c. False   d. True   e. False

55. a. True   b. True   c. True   d. True   e. False

56. a. True   b. True   c. True   d. True   e. False

57. a. False   b. True   c. True   d. True   e. True

58. a. False   b. False   c. False   d. True   e. True

Pleural effusion
Fluid which accumulates within the pleural cavity may be clear transudate, a serofibrinous or purulent exudates, hemorrhagic effusion or a chylous exudates. Causes are many:
- Inflammatory e.g. bacterial, pneumonia viral, tuberculosis, empyema.
- Neoplastic e.g. Bronchogenic cancer, Mesothelioma, Hodgkin's and metastatic disease.
- Others e. g. heart failure, Meigs syndrome, collagen disease, pericarditis pancreatitis, infarction, trauma, cirrhosis, others.

59. a. True   b. True   c. True   d. True   e. False

60. a. True   b. True   c. False   d. True   e. False

Wagner's Granulomatosis
Ulcerating necrotizing lesion of nasal passages associated with granulomatous pulmonary changes and occasionally glomerulonephritis.

Usually develop before the age of 40 years.

The pulmonary lesions are usually homogenous rounded opacities up to several centimeters in diameters simulating metastasis. The lesion may cavitate without surrounding infection. The granulomata may resolve in one area but subsequently develop in another zone.

Renal involvement is common and patient may have renal failure.

61. a. True   b. True   c. True   d. False   e. False

62. a. True   b. True   c. True   d. True   e. False

63. a. True   b. True   c. True   d. False   e. False

Miliary Tuberculosis
- Widespread haematogenous dissemination of Mycobacterium tuberculosis.
- So named because the nodules are the size of millet seeds (1–5 mm with mean of 2 mm).
- Miliary TB represents only 1–3% of all cases of TB.
- Older men, African Americans, and pregnant women are susceptible.
- Considered to be a manifestation of primary TB, although clinical appearance of miliary TB may not occur for many years after initial infection.
- When treated, clearing is frequently rapid. Miliary TB seldom, if ever, produces calcification.
- Under age 5, there is an increased risk of meningitis.

Risk Factors
- Immunosuppression, cancer, transplantation, HIV, malnutrition, diabetes, silicosis, end-stage renal disease.

Clinical Findings
- Onset is insidious.
- Patients may not be acutely ill.
- Symptoms include fever and weight loss, weakness and fatigue, chill, night sweats are common, cough, haemoptysis, anorexia.
- Hepatomegaly and lymphadenopathy are common.

Imaging Findings
- Takes weeks between the time of dissemination and the radiographic appearance of disease.
- Up to 30% have a normal chest radiograph.
- When first visible, they measure about 1 mm in size; they can grow to 2–3 mm if left untreated.
- Produces innumerable, non-calcified nodules.
- High resulotion CT scans are more sensitive at demonstrating small nodules.
- Nodules are either sharply or poorly defined, 1–4 mm in size.
- Diffused, random distribution.
- May be associated with interlobular septal thickening.
- If not treated, almost 100% fatal.
- With treatment, less than 10% mortality.

64. a. True   b. True   c. True   d. False   e. False

Atelectasis/Left Lower Lobe Atelectasis
- All types of atelectasis involve loss of volume in some or all of a lung with reluctant increased density of the involved lung.
- The atelectasis referred to her is that caused by bronchial obstruction, usually a tumour (i.e., a bronchogenic carcinoma), a foreign body, or a mucus plug.

Signs of Atelectasis
- Increase in density of the affected lung.
- Displacement of the fissure or the mediastinum towards the atelectasis.
- Crowding of the vessels and bronchial tree in the area of volume loss.
- Elevation of the hemidiaphragm.
- Overaeration of the opposite lung.

Imaging Signs of Left Lower Lobe Atelectasis
- Wedge-like density behind with base of triangle on the left hemidiaphragm and the apex at the hilum on frontal view.
- Silhouetting of all or just the medial portion of the left hemidiaphragm.
- Posterior displacement of the major fissure on the lateral view.
- Hilum may be displaced inferiorly.
- Descending branch of the pulmonary artery may disappear.
- There may be a spine sign due to superimposition of non-aerated lower lobe and the spine on the lateral view.
- In severe atelectasis of the lower lobe, the atelectasis lobe is so small it may not be recognisable on a conventional radiograph
    o The hemidiaphragm may be seen throughout its length, i.e., there is no silhouette sign.
    o The normal contour at the top left of the aortic knob may become invisible.
- Appearance of left lower lobe atelectasis is similar to right lower lobe atelectasis.

65. a. False   b. False   c. True   d. True   e. False

Hyaline membrane disease is a condition of unknown etiology. Affecting the premature infant especially those delivered by caesarean section or born of diabetic mothers. The alveoli are found to be lined by a thick Eosiphillic membrane that seriously interferes with gaseous exchange. The condition only occurs in the first few days of life.

Radiologically, widespread fine granular mottling that may produce a ground-glass appearance. Air bronchogram is commonly seen.

66. a. True   b. True   c. False   d. True   e. True

Primary Atypical Pneumonia (Mycoplasma Pneumoniae)
- Varied radiographically and clinically spread by direct contact/aerosol.
- Common in 5–20 years.
- Incubation period 1–2 weeks.
- Gradual onset beginning with pharyngitis, headache, myalgia.
- Dry cough, low fever, malaise, otitis, mild leukocytosis 20%.
- Most common respiratory cause of cold agglutinin production 60%.
- Pulmonary infiltrate, unilobar from hilum into lower lobe as earliest change 52%, bilobar 10%, atelectasis 29%.
- Consolidation in segmental lower lobe in 50%, bilateral 10–40%, pleural effusion 20%.

67. a. True   b. True   c. False   d. True   e. False

Bronchopulmonary Dysplasia (BPD)
- First described as a chronic lung disease seen in premature newborns treated for respiratory distress syndrome (RDS) with supplemental oxygen and mechanical ventilation for at least one week.
- It is now recognised that bronchopulmonary dysplasia (BPD) may complicate other types of neonatal lung disorders such as meconium aspiration syndrome and pneumonia.
- Common to almost all causes is oxygen administered under positive pressure.
- One definition involves an oxygen requirement at 28 days of life to maintain arterial oxygen tensions > 50 mm Hg accompanied by abnormal chest radiographs.

Clinical Findings
- Tachypnea and tachycardia, retractions, oxygen desaturation, weight loss.

Imaging Findings
- It may be impossible to distinguish the early stages of bronchopulmonary dysplasia from the later stages of respiratory distress syndrome (hyaline membrane disease).
- Coarse, irregular, rope-like, and linear densities represents atelectasis or fibrosis.
- Lucent, cyst-like foci; hyperexpanded areas of air-trapping.
- Hyperaeration of the lungs.
- Episodes of aspiration or pulmonary edema.
- Superimposed pneumonia.
- Pulmonary interstitial emphysema (PIE) may look identical, smaller air-containing spaces in PIE (bubbly appearance).

68. a. False   b. False   c. False   d. False   e. True

Pulmonary Alveolar Proteinosis (PAP)
General Considerations
- Rare disorder of unknown etiology.
- Alveoli are filled with PAS-positive proteinaceous material derived from surfactant phospholipids and proteins.
- Males are affected 4x more than females; the disease is most common from 20–50 years of age.
- It may be primary or secondary (to pulmonary infections, inhalation of silica or insecticides, and hematologic malignancies).
- Diagnosis is usually made by lung biopsy.

Clinical Findings
- Almost 1/3 may be asymptomatic even with abnormal chest radiographs.
- Symptoms, which are usually gradual in onset, include:
    o Dry cough (scant sputum production).
    o Progressive dyspnea.
    o Fatigue and malaise.
    o Weight loss.
    o Intermittent low-grade fever and/or night sweat.
    o Pleuritic chest pain.
    o Rarely cyanosis or haemoptysis.

Imaging Findings
- Bilateral perihilar consolidation in a configuration that may mimic pulmonary edema, but without cardiomegaly or pleural effusions.
- Occasional unilateral; lymphadenopathy is rare.
- Typically, changes progress over weeks to months into a diffuse reticulogranular pattern.
- On CT.
- Areas of patchy ground-glass opacification with smooth interlobular septal thickening and intralobular interstitial thickening → a polygonal pattern referred to as 'crazy paving'
    - DDX for 'crazy paving': exogenous lipoid pneumonia, Sarcoidosis, mucinous bronchoalveolar cell carcinoma, acute respiratory distress syndrome.

Differential Diagnosis
- Hypersensitivity pneumonitis
- Pneumocytosis Carinii pneumonia
- Pulmonary edema
- Sarcoidosis
- Lung cancer

69. a. False   b. True   c. True   d. True   e. True

Cavitary Pulmonary Metastases
- Metastases to the lung occur in about 30% of all malignant disease.
- Route of spread include haematogenous, lymphangitic, and direct extension.
- Most metastatic lung module develops through haematogenous spread.
- Primary lung carcinomas cavitate more frequently than metastatic lesions to the lung.
- Squamous cell carcinomas are the most common metastatic lesions to cavitate (70%) especially head and neck tumours.
- Pulmonary can rarely cavitate and almost always demonstrates associated adenopathy.
- Can be asymptomatic, especially slow-growing malignancies, e.g., papillary thyroid cancer or adenoid cystic carcinoma of the salivary gland.
- Later in course cancer is commonly dominated by sign and symptoms associated with primary tumour.

Imaging Findings
- Chest radiographs are usually first examination to detect pulmonary metastases.
- CT scanning has higher resolution than radiography, showing more smaller nodules.
- They are usually of differing sizes indicating different times of tumour embolization.
- They usually have thick and irregular walls.
- Metastases can be calcified, e.g., osteosarcoma, and can associated with pneumothorax.

70. a. True   b. True   c. False   d. False   e. False

Pulmonary Interstitial Emphysema
Abnormal location of pulmonary air within the interstitium and lyphatis secondary to barotrauma. Bubble-like or linear lucencies in the classic imaging.

71. a. False   b. False   c. False   d. False   e. True

Neonatal Pneumonia
Neonatal pneumonia – intrauterine infection or during delivery. Mostly group A beta nonhaemolytic streptococcus or E. coli.

Clinically marked respiratory distress, tachypnea, acidosis, septicemia, and shock. Patient not febrile.

Radiologically, perihilar streaky pattern may resemble transient tachypnea of newborn. Patchy air space disease, rarely pleural effusion. Lungs may stimulate hyaline membrane disease where diffuse homogenous infiltrates resembling ground-glass pattern.

72. a. True   b. True   c. True   d. False   e. True

Near drowning is aspiration due to after inhalation followed by survival a minimum of 24 hours.
After a forced expiration, an attempt at inspiration is made with closed mouth and nose. Whereby the negative pressure in the chest and lungs is made very subatmospheric, the reverse of Valsalva manoeuvre leads.

Near drowning is of several types and stages:
- Dry drowning seen in laryngospasm.
- In freshwater drowning hypervolemia.
- In seawater drowning hypovolemia.

Metabolic acidosis is seen in all types.

73. a. False   b. True   c. True   d. True   e. False

Histoplasmosis
- Endemic in South Africa, Southeast Asia, Central/North America, Ohio, Mississippi, St. Lawrence river valley and other.
- Spread by inhalation of wind-borne spores (microconida at 2-6 μm, macroconida at 6-8 μm) which germinate within alveoli releasing yeast torns.
- Pulmonary Histoplasmosis may be acute,if symptomatic, fever, cough, malise simulating viral upper respiratory infection 3 weeks after massive inoculums/debilitated patients (infants, elderly).
- Positive skin tests for Histoplasmosis, lymphadenopathy.
- Multiple nodules changing I to hundreds of punctuate calcification (usually 4 mm) after 9-24 months.
- Splenic calcification may occur.
- Histoplasmosis may be chronic, manifestation may be late, it may be disseminated.
- Chest radiograph may be normal however military/diffuse reticulonodular pattern rapidly progressing to diffuse air space opacification, hepatosplenomegaly and adenopathy may be present.

74. a. True   b. True   c. False   d. True   e. True

Skin Thickening of Breast

Normal skin thickness: 0.8-3 mm; may exceed 3 mm in inframammary region.

A. Localized skin thickening
- Trauma (prior biopsy), carcinoma, abscess, nonsuppurative mastitis and dermatologic conditions.

B. Generalized skin thickening.
- Skin is thickened initially and to the greatest extent in the lower dependent portion of breast.

- Overall increased density with coarse reticular pattern (= dilated lymph vessels + interstitial fluid triggering fibrosis).
  - a Axillary lymphatic obstruction
    1. Primary breast cancer = advanced breast cancer, invasive comedocarcinoma in large area, + primary breast cancer not necessarily seen due to small size/hidden location (axillary tail, behind nipple).
    2. Primary malignant lymphatic disease (e.g. lymphoma)
  - b Intradermal + inflammatory obstruction of lymph channels.
    1. Lymphatic spread of breast cancer from contralateral side.
    2. Inflammatory breast carcinoma = diffusely invasive ductal carcinoma.
  - c Mediastinal lymphatic blockage – Sarcoidosis, Hodgkin disease, advance bronchial/esophageal carcinoma and actinomycosis.
  - d Advanced gynecologic malignancies from thoracoepigastric collaterals – ovarian cancer and uterine cancer.
  - e Inflammation – acute mastitis, retromamillary abscess, fat necrosis, radiation therapy and reduction mammoplasty.
  - f Right heart failure – may be unilateral (R > L)
  - g Nephritic syndrome anasarca – dialysis and renal transplant.
  - h Subcutaneous extravasation following thoracocenthesis.

75. a. True   b. True   c. False   d. True   e. False

Metastasis to the lung occur in 30% of all malignancies, mostly haematogenous at any age likely after 50 years. Probability of pulmonary mets from kidney in 75%, osteosarcoma 75%, choriocarcinoma 75%, the thyroid, melanoma, and breast about 60%.

May be associated with pneumothorax especially in children with sarcoma.

Mets can be calcified especially from the breast, osteosarcoma, testes, thyroid (papillary), ovarian, or colon.
Mets can cavitate especially bronchogenic carcinoma, colon, melanoma, transitional cell carcinoma, etc.

76. a. True   b. False   c. True   d. False   e. True

Legionella pneumonia is caused by legionella pneumophilia transmission by direct inhalation, progressive respiratory failure, Hyponatremia, toxic encephalopathy may be present, can involve the liver, kidneys.

77. a. True   b. True   c. False   d. False   e. False

Bronchogenic Cyst (Foregut Duplication Cyst)
Developmental lesions that result from premature building of the tracheobronchial tree.

Appear as well-defined soft tissue mass. May identified incidentally or imaging studies. Almost always solitary not multilocular and not communicate with airway and do not contain air. Nay cause airway compression (mass effect).

Typically paratracheal, carinal, or hilar. Can involve the lung parenchyma.

Typically medial 1/3 of the lungs.

Typically not enhanced on CT scan. Wall enhancement may be seen with infection. Presence of air within the cyst may indicate infection.

78. a. True   b. True   c. True   d. True   e. False

79. a. False   b. True   c. True   d. True   e. False

Ground-Glass Opacity
In some patients with minimal interstitial disease, alveolitis, alveolar wall thickening, or minimal air space consolidation. A hazy increase in lung density can be observed on high resolution CT, which typically has patchy distribution. Ground-glass opacity is nonspecific and can be seen with variety of disease, e.g., viral pneumonia, pneumocystis carinii, edema, Desquamative interstitial pneumonitis, bronchiolitis, obliterans obstructing pneumonia, alveolar proteinosis, etc.

80. a. True   b. True   c. False   d. True   e. True

Others, e.g., hyaline membrane disease, Caplan's syndrome, chickenpox, pneumonia, siderosis others.

81. a. True   b. True   c. True   d. False   e. False

Also seen in neurofibromatosis, Goodpasture's syndrome, chemical inhalation, Sarcoidosis, tuberous sclerosis, lymphoma, leukaemia, tuberculosis, diffuse mycotic infections, and others.

82. a. True   b. True   c. False   d. False   e. True

Also seen in Sarcoidosis, pulmonary haemorrhage, rheumatic fever, pneumonia, drug hypersensitivity, idiopathic respiratory distress syndrome. Goodpasture's syndrome lymphoma, fat emboli, hyaline membrane disease, etc.

83. a. True   b. False   c. False   d. True   e. True

Also seen in tuberculosis, Sarcoidosis, scleroderma, neurofibromatosis, radiation, fibromatosis, rheumatic lung, tuberous sclerosis, etc.

84. a. True   b. True   c. True   d. True   e. False

85. a. True   b. True   c. False   d. False   e. False

Reactive Airways Disease
- General term for a disease usually in the paediatric featuring wheezing, shortness of breath, and coughing.
- Initial episodes are frequently referred to as bronchiolitis.
- Unlike asthma, which is chronic, reactive airways disease is usually transient although it can progress over time asthma.
- May be triggered by viral URIs, episode especially from respiratory syncytial virus (RSV), pollen and mold, cigarette smoke, and extreme cold.
- Most (60%) of children who have wheezing before age 3 will outgrow it by age 6.
- Use of the term is controversial; some believing it is too general.
- Increased respiratory rate, retractions, cough, fever, and Rhinorrhea.

Imaging Findings
- Peribronchial thickening.
    o Primary lobar or segmental bronchi.

- While the adults may have bronchi on end visible in the hila, children usually do not.
- Peribronchial thickening also produces tram-track like linear densities in the lung from bronchi visualise in profile.
- Hyperinflation.
- Atelectasis from mucus plugging.

Differential Diagnosis
- It is usually impossible to distinguish between viral bronchiolitis and asthma in a young child and the two coexist.
- Reactive airways dysfunction syndrome (RADS) and irritant-induced asthma (IrIA). Closely related forms of asthma that result from the nonimmulogic provocation of prolonged bronchial hyperresponsiveness and airflow obstruction by inhaled irritants.
- Anaphylactic reaction.
- Foreign body respiration.

86. a. True   b. False   c. False   d. True   e. True

87. a. True   b. True   c. True   d. False   e. True

88. a. False   b. True   c. True   d. True   e. True

89. a. True   b. True   c. True   d. False   e. True

Mediastinal Teratoma/Other Germ Cell Neoplasms
- Mediastinum is a rare site for occurrence of teratomas, most being ovarian in origin.
- Arise from primitive germ cell rests – supposed to migrate along urogenital ridge to primitive gonad; journey is interrupted in the mediastinum.
- May be solid or cystic – most are cystic.
- Three major categories:
  - Mature teratomas – well-defined from surrounding tissues; contain ectodermal elements along with cartilage, fat, and smooth muscle.
  - Immature teratomas – same elements as above with primitive tissues found in fetus.
  - Teratomas with malignant transformation – overall about 30% are malignant; usually adenocarcinoma in mature

teratomas; angiosarcoma or rhabdomyosarcoma in immature teratoma.
- Most of the cystic lesions are benign and most of the solid lesions are malignant.
- Both occur early in life – young adults most commonly.
- DDX from thymomas that usually occur in 5th or 6th decade.

Clinical Findings
- Usually asymptomatic.
- Large lesions can cause shortness of breath, cough, or retrosternal pain or fullness.
- Rare rupture of dermoid into trachea that leads to trichoptysis—expectoration of hair.

Associations
- Non-lymphocytic leukaemia and malignant Hystiocytosis with immature teratomas.

Imaging Findings
- Most occur in the anterior mediastinum, near junction of great vessels and heart.
- Benign lesions are usually smooth in contour whereas malignant masses ten to be lobulated.
- Usually larger than thymomas.
- Calcification may rarely occur but is no help since thymomas also calcify—exception would be the very rare occurrence of a tooth or bone in a dermoid.
- CT shows fatty mass with globular calcifications and rarely a tooth or a bone—fat-fluid level may be seen on CT.
- Rapid increase in size may mean haemorrhage in to a cyst rather than enlarging malignancy.

Treatment and Prognosis
- Mature teratomas – for benign cystic teratomas, surgical resection; excellent prognosis.
- Immature teratomas – in childhood, surgicalexcision is often successful; in adults, ten to have a more malignant course.
- Teratomas with malignancy – usually high aggressive; poor prognosis.

- Teratomas versus dermoid – dermoid only contain epidermis; teratomas contain all 3 germ layers, but are mostly endodermal when malignant.
- Other germ cell neoplasms – benign dermoid cysts; benign and malignant teratomas; seminomas; choriocarcinomas; embryonal cell carcinomas.

Mediastinal Seminomas
- Rare
- Almost always in young men
- Identical to testicular seminoma and ovarian dysgerminoma
- May be well-capsulated or invasive
- Tends to be lobulated
- Cannot be differentiated from teratoma

Primary Choriocarcinoma
- Even rare than seminoma in the mediastinum
- Only 23 reported in the literature, almost all in men
- Occur between 20–30 years
- May be lobulated
- May have elevated beta sub unit of HCG
- Growth is very rapid leading to dyspnea, haemoptysis, stridor
- Gynecomastia and A + Aschheim-Zondek test can occur
- Rapidly fatal

90. a. False   b. True   c. False   d. False   e. False

91. a. False   b. False c. True   d. False e. True

92. a. False   b. False c. False   d. False e. True

Tree-in-bud sign is a pattern describes the CT appearance of multiple area of centrilobular nodules with a linear branching pattern. Is a bronchioles filled with pus or inflammatory exudates, e.g., pulmonary tuberculosis or bronchiectasis with mucus plugging, e.g., cystic fibrosis or tumour emboli, e.g., breast cancer or as a result of bronchovascular interstitial infiltration, e.g., lymphoma, leukaemia, or as result of bronchiolitis, thickening of bronchial walls or bronvascular bundle, e.g., cytomegalovirus pneumonitis. Tree-in-bud sign is not visible on plain film. Usually seen in CT scan, best on HRCT.

Typically the centrilobular nodules are 2–4 mm in diameter and peripheral with 5 mm of pleural surface.

93. a. True   b. True   c. True   d. True   e. False

Accessory breast tissue can be found anywhere along the abdominal region of the milkline. Most frequently found in the axilla also found in chest wall, vulva, lateral thigh buttock, face ear, neck, knee. May be associated with hypertropic polyric stenosis testicular cancer patients are not aware of it till puberty response to hormonal stimulation and may become more evident during menarche, pregnancy, or lactation, supranumery nipples polyhelia may also present.

94. a. False   b. False   c. True   d. False   e. False

Pectus excavatum is depressed sternum seen in Marfan's syndrome can be diagnosed easily on chest x-ray. Swyer James-Macleod's syndrome is a rare lung condition that manifests as unilateral hemothorax lucency as result of post-infectious obliterative bronchiolitis.

95. a. True   b. True   c. True   d. True   e. False

96. a. True   b. True   c. True   d. True   e. False

Other complications: pulmonary hypertension, cyanosis, cor pulmonale.

97. a. True   b. False   c. False   d. False   e. True

98. a. True   b. True   c. True   d. True   e. False

Ellipsoid is wider than tall the sagittal and transverse dimension greater than anteroposterior dimension thin echogenic pseudocapsule is slow growing lesions. Hyperechogenicity is hyperechoic relative to subcutaneous fat in fibrous tissue speculation.

99. a. True   b. True   c. False   d. True   e. True

Benign ductal and stomal hyperplasia in the neonates and adolescents generally resolve on their own. May be associated with ACE inhibitors hormonal causes may require mastectomy.

Testicular ultrasound to role out hypogonadism.

100. a. True   b. True   c. True   d. False   e. True

101. a. True   b. True   c. False   d. False   e. False

Breast carcinoma is leading cause of death in women risk factors include old age, family history. Early menarche, late menopause, late first pregnancy, nulliparity lesions with suspicious imaging findings should be biopsied. On ultrasound, irregular heterogeneous hyperchoic mass. MRI ill-defined speculated and following contrast injection, it shows an initial rapid intense enhancement with a plateau on delayed scans secondary changes such as skin involvement nipple retraction, architectural distortion, can also be seen on MRI.

102. a. True   b. True   c. True   d. False   e. True

Asymptomatic palpable lump called breast mouse. Solid benign tumours with mixed epithelial and fibrous components seen from adolescence up to age 40 years. Malignancy occurring within fibro adenoma is very rare. On mammography, well-defined smoothly marginated lobulated ovoid lesions. Involuting fibro adenomas may show coarse 'pope-corn' calcifications on ultrasound. On an ultrasound mobile, often described as breast mouse. It is enhanced following gadolinium MRI.

103. a. False   b. True   c. True   d. True   e. True

Breast cyst is usually asymptomatic mass, and common may occur at any age. On mammography, occasionally wall calcification may be seen. On MRI, no solid component is seen in simple cysts following gadolinium. There is initial slow enhancement and persistent enhancement on delay images.

104. a. True   b. True   c. True   d. False   e. False

Flail chest – segment of thoracic cage is separated from reminder of chest wall by significant blunt chest trauma. Flail segment moves paradoxically with respiration. It moves inward on inspiration and outward on expiration.

Chest CT is invariably performed and may show rib fractures, pulmonary contusion, pulmonary laceration, pneumothorax, hemothorax, pneumomediastinum, subcutaneous emphysema, aortic injury, etc.

105. a. True   b. False   c. True   d. True   e. True

Irregular marginated tapering ends.

106. a. False   b. False   c. True   d. True   e. False

Seen also in pneumonia, lung cancer, breast cancer, asbestosis, sarcoidosis, pancreatitis, autoimmune disease especially rheumatoid arthritis, fungal infection, etc.

107. a. False   b. False   c. True   d. True   e. True

108. a. True   b. True   c. False   d. False   e. True

Transudate pleural effusion also seen in peritoneal dialysis, heart failure, cirrhosis, hypoalbuminaemia, constructive pericarditis.

109. a. False   b. False   c. True   d. True   e. False

Thymic sail sign is a normal appearance of thymus gland as it contacts minor fissure, while spinnaker sail sign is abnormal.

DiGeorge syndrome is hypoplasia of the thymus gland and parathyroids, with heart defects.

110. a. True   b. False   c. True   d. True   e. True

111. a. True   b. False   c. True   d. True   e. True

Medullary white pyramid sign of the kidney can be seen on unenhanced CT scan as high attenuation structures.

112. a. False   b. False   c. True   d. True   e. True

113. a. True   b. True   c. False   d. False   e. True

Air bronchogram is an aerated bronchi and bronchioles surrounded by confluent acinar atelectasis area.

114. a. True   b. False   c. True   d. False   e. True

115. a. True   b. False   c. True   d. True   e. True

116. a. False   b. True   c. True   d. True   e. True

Pneumatocele are intrapulmonary air-filled cystic spaces that can have a variety of sizes and appearances. Typically asymptomatic. They have thin wall and smooth inner margins.

117. a. True   b. False   c. True   d. False   e. True

118. a. False   b. True   c. False   d. True   e. False

In pleural effusion the trachea pushed away from the opacified side, so as in diaphragmatic hernia and any large mass.

The trachea pulled toward the opacified side in total lung collapse, pneumonectomy, and pulmonary hypoplasia.

The trachea remain central in consolidation pulmonary oedema, pleural mass, chest wall mass.

119. a. True   b. False   c. False   d. True   e. False

Usually occurs secondary to non-penetrating trauma.

Affect any age but children are considered more susceptible due to chest wall greater pliability in that age group.

The signs of contusion have often resolved properly.

Commonly occur in the lower lobes posteriorly.

120. a. False   b. True   c. True   d. True   e. True

121. a. False   b. True   c. True   d. True   e. True

122. a. True   b. True   c. True   d. False   e. True

1. The following are associated with pulmonary plethora and central cyanosis:
   a) Total anomalous P.V. drainage.
   b) Coronary artery arising from left main pulmonary artery.
   c) Ebstein anomaly.
   d) Pulmonary atresia.
   e) Truncus arteriosus.

2. In Epicardial fat pad the following are true:
   a) Seen in Cushing's syndrome.
   b) Can be mistaken with Morgagni hernia on conventional chest radiographs.
   c) It is normal.
   d) It is a lipoma.
   e) Enhances on CT scan.

3. The following are true in Abberent Right subclavian artery:
   a) May be presented with cough.
   b) May be presents with dysphagia lusoria.
   c) Most are asymptomatic.
   d) May be associated with cardiac defect.
   e) Associated with hiatal hernia.

4. In scimitar sign the following are true:
   a) Is an anomalous artery.
   b) Associated with dextrocardia.
   c) Causes a left to right shunt.

d) Causes central cyanosis.
   e) Associated with V.S.D.

5. In glomus tumour (hemangiopericytoma):
   a) Present with sharp pain exacerbates by slight trauma.
   b) Produces a well-defined dense bone lesion.
   c) The majority occur in the carpus.
   d) Are cured by adequate curettage.
   e) Associated with pulmonary AV anomalies.

6. The following cause pulmonary lesions, osseous lesions, and diabetes insipidus:
   a) Hystiocytosis.
   b) Sarcoidosis.
   c) Renal failure.
   d) Amyloidosis.
   e) Neurofibromatosis.

7. In truncus arteriosus the following are associated:
   a) Thymic agenesis.
   b) Right-sided aorta.
   c) Absent parathyroid gland.
   d) DiGeorge syndrome.
   e) Wide mediastinum shadow on plain radiograph.

8. In coarctation of the aorta:
   a) May be associated with Berry aneurysm.
   b) Is excluded if rib notching is unilateral.
   c) Hypertension is cured in 90% by surgery.
   d) May be associated with Turner's syndrome.
   e) May be associated with bicuspid valve.

9. In Eisenmenger syndrome following are true:
   a) The heart increases in size at the onset of reversed shunt.
   b) The plain chest radiogeph may be normal.
   c) First seen after 45 years and likely to be due to ASD.
   d) Calcification may be seen in pulmonary artery.
   e) Slow flow through the lungs is seen on pulmonary arteriography.

10. The causes of pulmonary hypertension are:
    a) Patent ductus arteriosus.
    b) Mitral incompetence.
    c) Kyphoscoliosis.
    d) Scimitar syndrome.
    e) Schistosomiasis.

11. Marfan's syndrome is associated with:
    a) Short patellar ligament.
    b) Aneurysm of the ascending aorta.
    c) Dextrocardia.
    d) Pes excavatum.
    e) Kyphoscoliosis.

12. Massive pulmonary oedema occurs in:
    a) Myocardial infarction.
    b) Ruptured ventricular septum.
    c) Ruptured chordal tendon.
    d) Post infarction syndrome.
    e) Traumatic fatty embolism.

13. Inferior vena cava thrombosis is associated with:
    a) Medial deviation of ureters.
    b) Increased presacral space.
    c) Splenomegaly.
    d) Bilateral renal enlargement.
    e) Can be diagnosed by CT angiogram.

14. In an abdominal aneurysm:
    a) 35% are above the renal vessels.
    b) Can be diagnosed by ultrasound.
    c) Gives pain in the back on palpation.
    d) Are excluded by a normal diameter aorta on aortography.
    e) A.P. plain film is the most suitable single film.

15. Upper lobe blood diversion occurs in:
    a) Mitral stenosis.
    b) Bilateral basal emphysema bullae.
    c) Valsalva manoeuvre.
    d) Pulmonary valvar stenosis.
    e) α 1 antitrypsin deficiency.

16. Turner's syndrome includes:
    a) Short metacarpal.
    b) Fused cervical vertebrae.
    c) Coarctation of aorta.
    d) Enlarged lateral femoral condyles.
    e) Enlarged adrenals.

17. In polycythemia Rubra Vera:
    a) There may be increase in white cell count and platelets.
    b) There is splenomegaly.
    c) Peptic ulcer is a recognised association.
    d) Renal vein thrombosis may occur.
    e) Erythrocyte sedimentation rate is high.

18. Accepted features of Fallot's tetralogy includes:
    a) Post stenotic dilatation of pulmonary artery.
    b) An enlarged right atrium.
    c) Enlarged descending aorta.
    d) Right-sided aortic arch.
    e) Plethoric lungs.

19. The following may be features of Marfan's disease:
    a) Atrial Septal Defect.
    b) Esophageal dilatation.
    c) Erosion of pituitary fossa.
    d) Dissecting aneurysm.
    e) Flat foot.

20. Small heart seen in:
    a) Emphysema.
    b) Constrictive pericarditis.
    c) Transposition of great vessels.
    d) Anorexia nervosa.
    e) Addison's disease.

21. Cyanotic congenital heart disease with increased pulmonary vascularity seen in:
    a) Eisenmenger physiology.
    b) Tricuspid atresia.
    c) Polysplenia.

d) Tetralogy of Fallot.
e) Common atrium.

22. Systemic hypertension may occur in:
    a) Addison's syndrome.
    b) Conn's syndrome.
    c) Neurofibromatosis.
    d) Subclavian steal syndrome.
    e) Adrenogenital syndrome.

23. Pulmonary stenosis occurs in:
    a) Mucopolysacharidosis I-H.
    b) Rubella syndrome.
    c) Turner's syndrome.
    d) Fallot's tetralogy.
    e) Noonan's syndrome.

24. Congestive heart failure may occur in neonates due to:
    a) Hyperglycaemia.
    b) Hyper ventilation.
    c) Aneurysm of vein of Galen.
    d) Haemangiomata of the liver.
    e) Raised intracranial pressure (ICP).

25. In Down syndrome:
    a) There is a decrease in the number of ossification centre in sternum.
    b) 11 pairs of ribs may be a feature.
    c) The most common cardiac abnormality is an endocardial cushion defect.
    d) There is an association with Hirschprung's disease.
    e) The hard palate is short.

26. Aortic regurgitation occur as a feature of:
    a) Reiter's syndrome.
    b) Homocystinuria.
    c) Idiopathic Hypercalcemia (William's syndrome).
    d) Marfan's syndrome.
    e) Ehlers-Danlos syndrome.

27. The following are true in pulmonary embolism;
    a) May have a normal chest x-ray.
    b) May be have a normal perfusion scan.
    c) The ventilation scan may be normal.
    d) Enhanced CT scan shows intraluminal lucencies in the pulmonary artery or its branches.
    e) Ascending phlebogram usually normal.

28. Fat emboli may give rise to:
    a) Pulmonary oedema.
    b) Usually pleural effusion.
    c) Petechiae.
    d) Cerebral symptoms.
    e) Sheehan's symptoms.

29. In cardiac pacemakers:
    a) Endocardiac electrode introduced through the subclavian vein.
    b) Ideally the tip of the electrode catheter should be situated in the apex of the right ventricle.
    c) The epicardial electrodes are usually introduced through the anterior chest wall.
    d) The epicardial electrodes must be fixed to the epicardium just behind the sternum.
    e) Position of electrodes are best checked by echocardiogram.

30. Unilateral rib notching is seen in:
    a) Coarctation of the oarta.
    b) Patent ductus arteriosus.
    c) Following a Blalock anastomosis.
    d) Neurofibromatosis.
    e) Myasthenia gravis.

31. In a patient with a ruptured aorta—the following are true:
    a) After blunt trauma, a widened mediastinum is diagnostic of aortic rupture.
    b) Rupture commonly occurs just beyond the left subclavian origin.
    c) Blurring of the aortic outline in an early sign.
    d) Lateral displacement of the superior vena cava is a sign of ascending aortic rupture.
    e) An intimal tear can be shown angiographically.

32. Pulmonary oedema commonly occurs in:
    a) Alveolar proteinosis.
    b) Heroin addiction.
    c) Gastric aspiration.
    d) Fallot's tetralogy.
    e) Multiple microemboli.

33. Pulmonary oedema in conjunction with a normal-size heart suggests:
    a) Myocardial infarction.
    b) Coarctation.
    c) Over transfusion.
    d) Acute glomerulonephritis.
    e) Aortic incompetence.

34. Septal lines (Kerley B Lines) are seen in:
    a) Infra cardiac TAPVD.
    b) Coal miners pneumoconiosis.
    c) Cryptogenic fibrosis.
    d) Due to dilated lymphatics.
    e) Sarcoidosis.

35. In anti trypsin deficiency:
    a) Upper lobe emphysema occurs.
    b) There is decreased flow to the low zones on isotope scan.
    c) Cor pulmonale develops very rarely.
    d) Associated with cirrhosis.
    e) Oesophageal varices.

36. The following cardiovascular conditions are contraindication in pregnancy:
    a) Marfan's syndrome.
    b) Severe obstructive valvular lesions.
    c) Severe pulmonary hypertension.
    d) Large secundum atrial septal defect with left to right shunt.
    e) Regurgitant lesions and left to right shunts without pulmonary hypertention.

37. Main pulmonary artery enlargement occurs in:
    a) Pulmonary stenosis.
    b) Pulmonary arterial hypertension.
    c) Pulmonary plethora.

d) Thymoma.
  e) Left to right shunt.

38. Pulmonary atresia:
    a) Is truncus arteriosus type 4.
    b) Absent pulmonary valve.
    c) Boot-shaped appearance of the heart.
    d) Large hilar shadow.
    e) Cardiac-gated T1W1: Pulmonary arteries best seen in axial and coronal planes.

39. Prominence of the ascending thoracic aorta likely seen:
    a) Aortic stenosis.
    b) Aortitis.
    c) Coarctation of aorta.
    d) Hypertension.
    e) Aortic insufficiency.

40. Causes of cardiomyopathy:
    a) Alcoholism.
    b) Diabetes insipidus.
    c) Collagen-vascular disease.
    d) Amyloidosis.
    e) Beri-beri.

41. Causes of pulmonary arterial hypertension are:
    a) Lung fibrosis.
    b) Arteritis.
    c) Multiple pulmonary emboli.
    d) High altitude.
    e) Thymoma.

42. Marked enlargement of cardiac silhouette:
    a) Cardiomyopathy.
    b) Pericardial effusion.
    c) Amyloidosis.
    d) Multiple valve disease.
    e) Coarctation of aorta.

43. The following are common on the right than the left side:
    a) Sequestrated lung segment.
    b) Pleural effusion associated with pancreatitis.
    c) Pleural effusion in Meig's syndrome.
    d) A ruptured hemidiaphragm following closed chest trauma.
    e) A Bochdalek hernia.

44. The following are true in acute chest syndrome (ACS):
    a) Clinical course is usually rapid.
    b) Pleural effusion or hemothorax are common.
    c) Blood and sputum cultures are frequently positive.
    d) Radiographs are abnormal at the start of an episode.
    e) On CT scan there may be ground-glass opacities in patchy, mosaic, or multifocal pattern of distribution.

45. Pulmonary sling are true:
    a) Distal trachea and carina often displaced to the left.
    b) The left pulmonary artery form a sling around the trachea as it passes leftward between the trachea and oesophagus.
    c) High position of the left hilum.
    d) Associated with dextrocardia.
    e) Incidence of pulmonary embolism is common.

46. In hypothyroidism:
    a) Psychosis.
    b) Increase cardiac pulsation.
    c) Anaemia.
    d) Carpal tunal syndrome.
    e) Hypothermia.

47. In postpericardiotomy syndrome (Dressler's syndrome):
    a) Symptoms typically appear 1–2 days following postcardiac injury syndrome.
    b) Leucopenia.
    c) Pleural effusion is rare.
    d) Parenchymal opacities are common.
    e) Pericardial effusion is common.

48. The following are true in pericardial effusion:
    a) Can be diagnosed confidently by conventional radiography.
    b) Echocardiogram is the study of choice.

c) CT scan can detect small effusion (less than 10 cc).
d) Collapse jugular veins are a feature.
e) Tamponade is commonly seen in association with pulmonary edema.

49. The common radiological abnormality in bird fancier's lung (pigeon) on CXR are:
    a) Pleural effusion.
    b) Lymphadenopathy.
    c) Progressive massive fibrosis (upper lobe shrinkage).
    d) Widespread bilateral micronodules opacities of soft tissue densities present.
    e) Cardiomegaly.

50. The following are true in meconium aspiration syndrome:
    a) Usually in premature infant.
    b) Collapsed lungs.
    c) Cyanosis.
    d) Brain damage.
    e) Air bronchogram on chest radiograph.

51. In superior mesenteric artery syndrome:
    a) Narrowing of angle between the aorta and superior mesenteric artery.
    b) Seen in those with asthenic build.
    c) Associated with aortic aneurysm.
    d) On barium meal megaduodenum is present.
    e) Associated with pyloric stenosis.

52. Tetany is recognised feature in:
    a) Asthma.
    b) Hyperventilation.
    c) Pyloric stenosis.
    d) Malabsorption syndrome.
    e) Anorexia nervosa.

53. The following are common in septic pulmonary emboli:
    a) Pleural effusion.
    b) Bilateral emphysema.
    c) Pneumothorax.

d) Bilateral Hilar-lymphadenopathy.
   e) Empyema.
54. Rib notching in coarctation of the aorta:
   a) Most often involve 4th–8th rib inclusive on both sides.
   b) Isolated right-sided notching occurs when left subclavian artery is involved in actual coarctation.
   c) Can be seen in infants and childhood on chest radiograph.
   d) Is due to dilated intercostals arteries.
   e) The superior margin of the ribs are the likely involved part.

55. In aortic dissection:
   a) More in male over 40 years.
   b) Hypertension is the most common predisposing factors.
   c) Right pleural effusion with mediastinal widening on plain radiograph is a feature.
   d) Asymmetric peripheral pulses.
   e) Left paraspinal stripe on plain radiograph.

56. The azygos vein is often enlarged in:
   a) Lymphageiectasis.
   b) Absence of inferior vena cava.
   c) Pregnancy.
   d) Pulmonary edema from heart failure.
   e) Carcinoma of bronchus.

57. In femoral artery pseudoaneurysm (false aneurysm):
   a) Always associated with a history of blunt or penetrating trauma.
   b) Typical presentation includes pain, swelling, and palpable mass in the groin.
   c) Conservative management is the first-line treatment of false aneurysm.
   d) Groin mass maybe pulsatile or have a bruit or thrill, which demonstrates flow within the mass.
   e) On color Doppler ultrasound the blood flow has a characteristic 'yin-yang' appearance rapidly filling and swirling during systole and emptying during diastole.

58. Causes of pericardial effusion:
   a) Tuberculosis.
   b) Histoplasmosis.
   c) Lupus erythromatosis.

d) Hyperparathyroidism.
e) Alcoholism.

59. Tuberous sclerosis is associated with;
    a) Angiomyolipoma of the kidney.
    b) Rhabdomyomas of the heart.
    c) Retinal phacoma.
    d) Recurrent pneumothorax.
    e) Exclusively in male.

60. The following are most common:
    a) Primary tumour of heart in child rhabdomyoma.
    b) Primary benign heart tumour in myxoma.
    c) Cardiac tumour in metastatic disease, e.g., melanoma.
    d) Type 1 of TAPVR is supracardiac.
    e) Right to left shunt in atrial septal defect.

61. Cyanosis with decreased vascularity of the lung seen in:
    a) Tetralogy.
    b) Truncus-type IV.
    c) Tricuspid atresia.
    d) Transposition.
    e) Congenital mitral stenosis.

62. Causes of congestive heart failure are:
    a) Fluid overload.
    b) Right to left shunts.
    c) Mitral stenosis.
    d) Hypertension.
    e) Coronary artery disease.

63. Permanent absent of the thymus shadow occur in:
    a) Steroid's therapy in Addison's disease.
    b) Dysgammaglobulinemia.
    c) DiGeorge syndrome.
    d) Burned baby.
    e) Complete transportation of great vessel.

64. Causes of enlarged main pulmonary artery are:
    a) Pulmonary stenosis.
    b) Right to left shunt.

c) Left to right shunt.
d) Idiopathic.
e) Pulmonary venous hypertention.

65. Causes of venous pulmonary hypertention are:
    a) TAPVR from below diaphragm.
    b) Right atrial myxoma.
    c) Cor triatria.
    d) Congenital mitral stenosis.
    e) Coarctation of aorta.

66. Causes of prominence of entire thoracic aorta are:
    a) Aortic stenosis.
    b) Co-arctation of the aorta.
    c) Hypertension.
    d) Aortic insufficiency.
    e) Atherosclerosis.

67. Causes of enlarged left atrium are:
    a) Mitral regurgitation.
    b) Prolapsed mitral valve.
    c) Right atrial myxoma.
    d) Congestive heart failure.
    e) Papillary muscle dysfunction.

68. Radiographic features of tuberous sclerosis are:
    a) Cardiac rhabdomyomas.
    b) Renal angiomyolipoma (AML).
    c) Lymphangiomyomatosis (LAM).
    d) Facial angiofibromas.
    e) Multiple meningioma.

69. Predisposed conditions to septic emboli are:
    a) Alcoholism.
    b) Tricuspid valve endocarditis.
    c) Carbuncles.
    d) Pelvic lipomatosis.
    e) Pelvic thrombophlebitis.

70. In cardic myxoma:
    a) The most common primary cardiac tumour in adults.
    b) May be found incidentally on imaging of the heart.
    c) Commonly arising from the ventricles.
    d) On CT scan usually heterogeneously low attenuating mass.
    e) T1 c+ (Gd) show enhancement on MRI.

71. In calcification of left atrium:
    a) Almost always associated with rheumatic mitral stenosis.
    b) Almost always associated with atrial fibrillation.
    c) Almost always associated with thrombus in the appendage.
    d) Almost always involve the interatrial septum.
    e) Massive calcification of the left atrial walls called porcelain atrium.

72. A 30-year-old short status male presented with sudden chest pain, on examination he has low-set ears, low hairline, hearing loss. The following are likely diagnosis:
    a) Marfan's syndrome.
    b) Turner's syndrome.
    c) Alkapton uria (ochronotic arthritis).
    d) Osteopetrosis (marble bones).
    e) Achondroplasia.

73. There is a recognised association between oral contraceptives and:
    a) Reduced risk of ovarian and endometrial cancer.
    b) Benign hepatic adenoma.
    c) Focal nodular hyperplasia of the liver.
    d) Mesenteric vein thrombosis.
    e) Crohn's disease.

74. Which of the following statements are true:
    a) Pulmonary embolism is more frequent on the left side than the right side.
    b) Fracture of an upper rib is a common accompaniment of traumatic bronchial laceration.
    c) The radiological changes of pulmonary contusion occur within 12 hours of the initiating trauma.
    d) Following blunt chest injury a normal chest radiograph excludes aortic rupture.
    e) Air crescent sign on chest x-ray and CT scan classically in aspergillomas.

75. The following are associated with congenital heart disease:
    a) Hypertrophic pulmonary osteoarthropathy.
    b) Triphalangeal thumb.
    c) Carpal fusion.
    d) Scoliosis.
    e) Acromegalic mother.

76. The following may be associated with hypothyroidism:
    a) Enlarged heart.
    b) High output cardiac failure.
    c) Pericardial effusion.
    d) The heart may return to normal without treatment.
    e) Dermatographia.

77. Turner's syndrome is associated with:
    a) Low-set ear.
    b) Low hair line.
    c) Bicuspid aortic valve.
    d) Tall status.
    e) Glaucoma.

78. In kawasaki disease (mucocutaneous lymph node syndrome):
    a) Acute systemic vasculitis affecting small- and medium-sized arteries.
    b) Multiple coronary aneurysms.
    c) Can be diagnosed confidently by echocardiography.
    d) Self-limiting disease in the majority of cases.
    e) Associated with Takayasu's disease.

79. Plethoric lungs fields are seen in conditions that increase pulmonary blood flow:
    a) Transposition of great arteries with ASD or VSD.
    b) Truncus arteriosus.
    c) Left to right shunt (ASD, VSD, PDA) coronary artery fistula into right heart, aortopulmonary window.
    d) Total anomalous pulmonary venous connection.
    e) Ebstein's condition.

80. In aortic arch:
    a) It may be on the right side.
    b) It may be double.

c) Bovine arch is commonly seen in African descent.
d) Thyroidea in an artery is a branch of the arch.
e) Terminate at the lower border of thoracic 6 vertebras where it continues as the descending aorta.

81. D-transposition the following are true:
a) Aorta arises from right ventricle.
b) Pulmonary artery arises from the left ventricle.
c) 'Egg-on-side' cardiomediastinal silhouette on plain film.
d) Oligemic lungs.
e) Wide mediastinum on plain radiography.

82. The following signs maybe seen in pulmonary embolism on plain radiograph or CT scan:
a) Dense hilum sign.
b) Comet tail sign.
c) Air crescent sign.
d) Knuckle sign.
e) Hampton's hump sign.

83. In vascular calcification:
a) Maffucci's syndrome.
b) Milk-alkali syndrome
c) Werner's syndrome.
d) Immobilisation syndrome.
e) Down syndrome.

84. In DiGeorge syndrome 'relocardiofacial syndrome':
a) Associated with truncus arteriosus.
b) Associated with tetralogy of Fallot.
c) Increase risk of schizophrenia.
d) Cleft palate.
e) Hypercalcemia.

85. In endomyocardial fibrosis:
a) Young male Africans are commonly affected.
b) Gross enlargement of both side of the heart.
c) Universally fatal.
d) Pericardial effusion is rare.
e) Severe mitral valve incompetence and tricuspid incompetence are present.

86. In endocardial fibroelastosis:
    a) Elderly females are commonly affected.
    b) Marked myocardial insufficiency.
    c) Pulmonary edema and heart failure are common.
    d) Endocardiac calcification.
    e) Fluoroscopy shows marked diminished cardiac pulsation.

87. Classical chest radiograph in mitral stenosis are:
    a) Double right heart border.
    b) Small pulmonary artery.
    c) Cardiomegaly.
    d) Prominent left atrial appendage.
    e) Splaying of the subcarinal angle.

1. a. True   b. True   c. False   d. False   e. False

Central cyanosis is often due to a circulatory or ventilator problem that leads to poor blood oxygenation in the lungs. It develops when arterial saturation drops to < 85%.

Acute cyanosis may be due to the following causes:
1. Central nervous system (impairing normal ventilation) e.g. intracranial haemorrhage or drugs (Heroin) or seizures.
2. Respiratory system e. g. bronchospasm (asthma) or pulmonary embolism, pulmonary hypertension, inflammatory lungs & bronchiolitis.
3. Cardiac disorder e.g. tetralogy of fallot, right to left shunts, heart failure, myocardial infarction
4. Blood, polycythemia, methenoglobinemia.
5. Others, e.g. high altitude, hypothermia, obstructive sleep apnea.

2. a. True   b. True   c. True   d. False   e. False

Epicardial (Pericardial) Fat Pad
- An accumulation of fat between the parietal pericardium and the parietal pleura, usually found incidentally on chest radiography.
- Most common either the right cardiophrenic or adherent to the left ventricle at the apex of the heart.
    o On the left side, it blunts the normal rounded apex of the heart.
- May also become larger in mediastinal lipomatosis caused by Cushing syndrome or exogenous steroid administration.

- 'Mass' of fat density that does not silhouette the adjacent soft tissue of the heart or diaphragm, usually seen best on frontal radiographs.
- Low Hounsfield (negative) numbers on CT.

Differential Diagnosis
- Morgagni hernia.
- Pericardial cyst.
- Incidental finding requiring no treatment.

3. a. True   b. True   c. True   d. True   e. False

The Aberrent Right Subclavian Artery (ARSA) arises as last branch from the aortic arch. Occurs less than 1% of people. It passes trachea and oesophagus forward. Produce oblique shadow above aortic arch on frontal film. The origin of ARSA may be dilated. Most are asymptomatic, may cause encircling vascular ring-like pulmonary sling. May produce dysphagia (dysphagia lusoria) on barium swallow frontal view in half-filled oesophagus, just below aortic knuckle may see on long length oblique impression of the oesophagus.

4. a. False   b. True   c. True   d. False   e. True

Scimitar syndrome – Partial anomalous pulmonary venous return, associated with hypogenetic lung. The anomalous vein has morphology of scimitar (sword).
- Drain below the level of diaphragm into the level of I.V.C. or portal vein
- Associated with accessory diaphragm (diaphragmatic hernia).
- Also associated with hemivertebra rib notching, ASD, VSD, and PDA, dextra position of the heart.
- There is no central cyanosis.

5. a. True   b. False   c. False   d. True   e. False

Glomus jugulare tumours (Hemangiopericytoma) – highly differentiated benign vascular neoplasm affect soft tissue more than bone. Women are more commonly affected. Commonly affects the terminal phalanges of the fingers. May resemble an aneurysmal bone cyst or chondroma. May cause episodes of stabbing pain over some years. Excision provides complete relief of pain. Can rise in the region of the jugular bulb and extend into the petrous bone and internal ear and producing basal erosion.

6.   a. True   b. True   c. True   d. False   e. True

Diabetes insipidus is excessive urination and extreme thirst as a result of inadequate output of the pituitary hormone, ADH (Antidiuretic hormone also called vasopressin), or lack of the normal response by the kidney to ADH.

Types are central and nephrogenic, some can involve the pulmonary condition.

Skeleton systems are associated with diabetes insipidus including Sarcoidosis, tuberculosis, tuberous sclerosis, neurofibromatosis, chronic nephritis.

7.   a. True   b. True   c. True   d. True   e. False

Truncus Arteriosus (Common Arterial Trunk) common arterial vessel arises from the heart giving rise to aorta, pulmonary arteries, and common arteries. Most commonly associated with right aortic arch, absent thymus, absent parathyroid glands (neonatal tetany), DiGeorge syndrome.

Patient is cyanotic, cardiomegaly increased pulmonary vascularity, narrow mediastrium.

8.   a. True   b. False   c. True   d. True   e. True

Coarctation of the aorta – classical coartation occurs in the juxtra-ductal position. It presents most frequently in adult life with hypertension. (However, a small group present is the neonatal period with left heart failure.) Berry aneurysms in the brain are extremely serious because they can rupture or leak and cause strokes or they can be fatal.

Turner's syndrome, which is confined to females, is associated with congenital cardiac and aortic lesion and anomalies of the kidneys such as malrotation.

Typical rib notching on lower border of fourth to eight ribs, most marked in the mid-third of the posterior rib projection. There are several causes of rib notch, e.g., neurofibromatosis, subclavian obstruction, pulmonary oligaemia.

9. a. False   b. False   c. False   d. True   e. True

Eisenmenger reaction is where there is right to left shunt associated with a well-elevated pulmonary vascular resistance, will lead to radiological appearance of clearly variable pulmonary oligaema. However, the main pulmonary artery enlarged and its main branches. Calcification can be seen in those patients in athermanous plaques or mural thrombi in the main pulmonary arteries. Hyperkinetic circulation pulmonary angiography is a method of study.

10. a. True   b. True   c. True   d. False   e. True

Pulmonary hypertension present either the pulmonary arterial or pulmonary venous pressure is elevated their normal level and the problem must be considered under those two headings, arterial and venous
The causes are many including hyperdynamic e.g. left-right shunt in ASD, VSD, PDA and TAPVD. It may be obstructive in pulmonary venous hypertension in MS, MI, atrial myxoma contratrium.

Vasoconstriction secondary to hypoxia in case of high altitude, chronic bronchitis, kyphoscoliosis or upper respiratory tract obstruction.

Pulmonary hypertension is also seen in obliterative condition e.g. arteritis, schistosomiasis or thrombi and emboli.

Scimitar syndrome in which part of the right pulmonary venous blood return to inferior vena cava.

11. a. False   b. True   c. False   d. True   e. True

Marfan's Syndrome (Arachnodactyly)
Tall thin structure with long limbs arm span greater than height. Hypotonicity, elongated face, high arch palate. Elongation of phalanges and metacarpals, metacarpal index (averaging the 4 ratio of the length of 2nd through 5th divided by their respective mid diaphyseal width).

Clubfoot, hallux valgus, hypermobility of joints, pectus excavatum, kyphoscoliosis, winged scapula, recurrent dislocation of the patella, hip, clavicle, and mandible. Elbow increase interpedicular distance.

12. a. True b. True c. True d. False e. False

Pulmonary Oedema
Accumulation of excessive fluid in interstitial spaces of lung with subsequent movement of fluid into the pulmonary alveolar spaces. Fluid accumulation is due to imbalance between rate of production and removal.

Causes are many, aspirations, e.g., Mandelson's syndrome, cerebral (stroke, head trauma, epilypsy) shock (e.g., insulin reaction, shock therapy), thoracic trauma, nephritis, narcosis, transfusion reaction, cardiomyopathy, heart disease.

Oxygen toxicity – fluid overload, high altitude, hypoproteinemia, mediastinal disease with venous or lymphatic obstruction, pregnancy, suffocation, and others.

13. a. False b. True c. True d. True e. True

Inferior Vena Cava Thrombosis
The clinical presentation depend on extend and location of thrombus. Thrombophilic screening and evaluation of the clotting and fibrinolytic systems may aid in the diagnosis of this condition.

Contrast renography remains the criterion standard as the optional diagnostic study for inferior vena cava thrombosis.

Medical management focuses on anticoagulant and thrombolytic therapy.

Surgical management consists of caval interruption, thrombectomy, or endovascular interventions.

14. a. False b. True c. True d. False e. False

Abdominal aortic aneurysm ballooning focal widening of abdominal aorta > 3 cm (by ultrasound). Twice the size of normal aorta (> 4 cm). Commonly male >75 years; white > blacks.

Hypertension, cigarette smoking, family history, hypercholesterolemia. About 90% of abdominal aortic aneurysm occurs infra renal. Can extend to include one or both of the iliac arteries in the pelvis. Lateral view of the abdomen is the most suitable single film.

15. a. True   b. True   c. False   d. False   e. True

16. a. True   b. False   c. True   d. False   e. False

17. a. True   b. True   c. True   d. True   e. False

18. a. False   b. False   c. False   d. True   e. False

19. a. True   b. True   c. False   d. True   e. False

20. a. True   b. True   c. False   d. True   e. True

21. a. False   b. True   c. False   d. False   e. True

22. a. False   b. True   c. True   d. False   e. True

23. a. False   b. True   c. True   d. True   e. True

24. a. False   b. False   c. True   d. True   e. True

25. a. False   b. True   c. True   d. True   e. False

26. a. True   b. False   c. False   d. True   e. True

27. a. True   b. True   c. True   d. True   e. False

28. a. True   b. False   c. True   d. True   e. False

29. a. True   b. True   c. True   d. True   e. False

30. a. True   b. False   c. True   d. True   e. False

31. a. True   b. True   c. False   d. True   e. True

32. a. False   b. True   c. False   d. False   e. False

33. a. True   b. False   c. True   d. True   e. False

34. a. True   b. True   c. True   d. False   e. True

35. a. False   b. True   c. False   d. True   e. True

36. a. False   b. False   c. False   d. True   e. False

37. a. True   b. True   c. True   d. False   e. True

38. a. True   b. True   c. True   d. False   e. True

39. a. True   b. True   c. True   d. False   e. False

40. a. True   b. False   c. True   d. True   e. True

41. a. True   b. True   c. True   d. True   e. False

42. a. True   b. True   c. True   d. True   e. False

43. a. False   b. False   c. True   d. False   e. True

44. a. True   b. False   c. False   d. False   e. True

Acute Chest Syndrome (ACS)
- Leading causes of death amongst patients with sickle cell anaemia.
- Syndrome is characterised by new air spaces disease on chest x-ray, and one or more of the following such as fever (variable), cough, sputum production, shortness of breath, hypoxia.
- Exact cause is unknown.
- Most often affects those with homozygous sickle cell and sickle cell-beta thalassemia genotypes.
- More common in the winter, in younger individuals, and after surgery.
- More severe in adolescent and adults (> 20) than in children.
- May be recurrent.
- Clinical course is usually rapid.
- Symptoms can range from mild to fatal.
- Blood and sputum cultures are frequently negative.
- There may be chest wall tenderness from rib infarctions.

Imaging Findings
- Pathogenesis of all the air space disease in ACS is not fully understood. Part of it is commonly caused by non-embolic thrombosis of sickled erythrocytes in the pulmonary vasculature.
- Radiographs may be normal at the start of an episode.
- On conventional radiographs, patchy airspace disease in a segmental, lobar, or multilobar distribution and may or may not have a pleural effusion.
- Airspace disease may also be made up of atelectasis, pneumonia, or fat embolism. Fat embolism occurs from bone marrow necrosis and is thought by some to play a key role in the pathogenesis of the syndrome.
- On CT, there may be ground-glass opacities in a patchy, mosaic or multifocal pattern of distribution.

45. a. True   b. True   c. False   d. False   e. False

Pulmonary Sling
Anomalous origin of the pulmonary artery. The left pulmonary artery arises from the right pulmonary artery forms a sling around the trachea as it passes leftward between the trachea and eosophagus.
Typically presents early in the life with severe stridor. May be associated with complete tracheal rings. Low position of the hilum on radiography. Tracheal compression typically best demonstrated on axial CT or MRI.

46. a. True   b. False   c. True   d. True   e. True

Hypothyroidism (Myxodema / Mucoprotein Accumulation)
- Causes primary autoimmune thyroiditis, Hashimoto's disease. Pituitary failure prolongs iodine deficiency. Antithyroid drugs inherited enzyme defects, thyroidectomy, or radioactive iodine therapy.
- Radiologically, cardiomegaly however the heart returns to normal after treatment. Diminish cardiac pulsation on fluoroscopy. Small cardiac effusion may be seen.

47. a. False   b. False   c. False   d. True   e. True

Postpericardiotomy Syndrome / Dressler's Syndrome / Postmyocardial Infarction Syndrome / Postcardiac Injury Syndrome

- Autoimmune and febrile illness that can follow coronary artery bypass surgery.
- May also be seen following myocardial infarction (Dressler's syndrome).
- Occur in 10–40% of cases.
- Combination of pericarditis, pleuritis, and pneumonitis.
- Symptoms typically appear 2–3 weeks following infarct/surgery—sometimes years.
- Pleuritic chest pain (91%), fever, pericardial, and pleural effusion; pericardial friction rub, effusions can be bloody and cause tamponade, shortness of breath, leukocytosis.

Diagnosis can be usually be made from a combination of the clinical picture and chest radiographs (95% abnormal).

Cardiac silhouette enlargement from pericardial effusion and mild to moderate-sized, pleural effusion may be bilateral.
- Pleural effusions (80%)
- Parenchymal opacities (75%)
- Enlarged cardiac silhouette from pericardial effusion (50%)

Differential Diagnosis
Different from more common post myocardial infarction reactive changes occurs between days 2 and 4 after the infarction, congestive heart failure, pneumonia, reaction to medication.

48. a. True   b. True   c. False   d. False   e. False

Pericardial Effusion
Abnormal amount of fluid in the pericardial space, defined as the space between the visceral and parietal layers of the pericardium. Normally contains about 20–50 cc of fluid. Fat covers outside of heart and outside of pericardium sandwiching pericardial space between the two layers. Normal thickness of pericardium (parietal pericardium and fluid in space) is 2–4 mm.

Small effusions frequently produce no symptoms. Chest pain or discomfort with a characteristic of being relieved by sitting up or leaning forward and worsened in the supine position. Syncope, palpitations, shortness of breath, tachypnea. Muffled or distant heart sounds, tachycardia; hypotension; jugular venous distension. Pulsus paradoxus decrease in systolic pressure with inspiration of more than 10 mm Hg. Rate of accumulation of fluid is proportional to severity of symptoms, the faster the fluid accumulates, the more severe the symptoms.

Requires about 150–250 cc before cardiac tamponade occurs about 7–10% of those with pericardial effusion are at risk for developing tamponade; tamponade compresses heart and causes low cardiac output; most effusions do not lead to cardiac tamponade; size of cardiac silhouette is frequently increased; tamponade is rarely seen in association with pulmonary edema in the lungs.

Causes of Pericardial Effusions
1. Myocardial infarction.
2. Collagen vascular disease.
3. Trauma.
4. Metastatic disease.
5. Tuberculosis.
6. Viral infection.
7. Uremia.

Conventional Radiography
Suggestive but not usually diagnostic, 'water bottle configuration' is symmetrically enlarged cardiac silhouette, loss of retrosternal clear space, rapidly enlarging cardiac silhouette with nornmal pulmonary vascularity.

Echocardiogram
Study of choice, echo-free fluid between the visceral and parietal pericardium, early effusions accumulate posteriorly first, > 1 cm is usually defined as a 'large' effusion.

CT
May detect small effusions (50 cc), fluid-filled space surrounding the myocardium, early effusions accumulate posteriorly first.

49. a. False   b. False   c. True   d. True   e. False

Pigeon Fancier's Disease and Budgerigar Fancier's Disease
Pigeon fancier's disease is type of extrinsic allergic alveolitis due to inhalation of antigens.

In acute stage, fine soft tissue shadows may be present but ground-glass appearance all over the lungs is common.

They are usually basal but can disappear after removal from contact.

Late stage pulmonary fibrosis and bullae, however nodular opacities may persist with fibrosis, Broncheictasis, and emphysematous lung.

50. a. False   b. False   c. True   d. True   e. False

Meconium Aspiration Syndrome
- Most common cause of neonatal respiratory distress in full-term/postmature infants.
- Meconium in amniotic fluid of about 20% of pregnancies.
- Meconium products produce bronchial obstruction and air trapping. Chemical pneumonitis takes place.
- The respiratory distress more severe than transient tachypnea of the newborn and happen immediately.
- On the chest radiograph, hyperinflation of both lungs, diffuse densities, spontaneous pneumothorax, and pneumomediastinum. Pleural effusion may be present. No air bronchogram. Cyanosis or anoxic brain damage may happen, pulmonary hypertension, and right to left shunting is a complication.

51. a. True   b. True   c. False   d. True   e. False

Superior Mesenteric Artery Syndrome
- Compression of 3rd portion of duodenum between the aorta and superior mesenteric artery (SMA). Patient presented with epigastric pain, nausea, abdominal cramping and repeated vomiting.
- Typically findings are worst in supine position and may be relieved by changing to the prone or left lateral decubitus positions.
- Usually requires upper G.I. or C.T. of abdomen for diagnosis.
- Vertical linear compression defect in transverse portion of duodenum overlying spine.
- Abrupt change in caliber distal to compression defect treated surgically.

52. a. False   b. True   c. True   d. True   e. True

Tetany an abnormal condition characterised by periodic painful muscular spasm and tremors caused by faulty calcium metabolism and associated with diminished function of the parathyroid glands.

53. a. False   b. False   c. False   d. False   e. True

Septic Pulmonary Emboli
- Majority: < 40 years old.

Predisposing Factors
- IV drug abusers
- Alcoholism
- Immunodeficiency
- Heart diseases
- Dermal infection

Sources
- Tricuspid valve endocarditis

Most common in IV drug abusers
- Pelvic thrombophlebitis, infected venous catheter or pacemaker wire, arteriovenous shunts for hemodialysis, drug abuse producing septic thrombophlebitis (e.g. heroin addicts), peritonsillar abscess, and osteomyelitis.

Organism
- S. Aureus, streptococcus

Clinical finding
- Sepsis, cough, dyspnea, haemoptysis, chest pain, high fever, shaking/chills, severe sinus tachycardia, and lung abscess.

Chest radiograph shows multiple round or wedge-shaped densities, cavitation, frequently thin walled migratory old ones and new ones. Pleural effusion is rare.

Hilar and mediastinal adenopathy can occur on CT scan, multiple peripheral parandymal nodules. Cavitation or air bronchogram more than 80%. Cavitation with walled and may have no fluid level. Wedge-shaped subpleural lesion with apex of lesion directed toward pulmonary hilum.

Feeding vessels sign the pulmonary artery leading to nodule > 60%.

The differential diagnosis is rheumatoid nodules, squamous, or transitional cell metastases. Necrotizing granulomatosis, empyema is common complication.

54. a. True   b. True   c. False   d. True   e. False

By far, the most frequent cause of rib notching is co-arctation of the aortic arch. Rib notching is not usually present in the infant or child with co-arctation. It generally becomes evident in the adolescent years. The notching in co-arctation is due to the dilated tortuous intercostals arteries carrying blood from the dilated collateral vessels to the dorsal aorta distal to the narrowing. Thus the normal blood flow in these intercostals is reversed. The indentations are sited on the middle third and on the under border of the ribs.

55. a. True   b. True   c. False   d. True   e. True

Aortic Dissection
- Haemorrhage in the media (at vasa vasorum) leading to either haemorrhage in separate media from adventitia or leading to haemorrhage in the wall (less common).
- Hypertension is most common predisposing factor however atherosclerosis, Marfan's syndrome, coarctation of oarta, aortic stenosis, etc.
- The size of the ascending aorta > 5 cm and descending aorta > 4 cm. When the ascending aorta involve (standford type A) when the ascending aorta is not involve (standford type B).
- Chest film may shows left pleural effusion.
- MRI is best for imaging ascending aorta.
- Contrast enhanced CT scan image arch and descending aorta.
- Angiography for intimal flap, double lumen, aortic wall thickness > 10 mm, obstruction of branch vessels, etc.

56. a. False   b. True   c. True   d. True   e. True

- Also seen in constrictive pericarditis portal hypertension, aorto-azygous fistula, pericardial effusion, tricuspid insufficiency, etc.

57. a. True   b. True   c. False   d. True   e. True

58.	a. True	b. True	c. True	d. False	e. False
59.	a. True	b. True	c. True	d. True	e. False
60.	a. True	b. True	c. True	d. True	e. False
61.	a. True	b. True	c. True	d. True	e. False
62.	a. True	b. False	c. True	d. True	e. True
63.	a. False	b. False	c. True	d. False	e. True
64.	a. True	b. False	c. True	d. True	e. False
65.	a. True	b. False	c. True	d. True	e. True
66.	a. False	b. False	c. True	d. True	e. True
67.	a. True	b. True	c. False	d. True	e. True
68.	a. True	b. True	c. True	d. True	e. False

Classically described as presenting in childhood with a triad of:
1. Seizures
2. Mental retardation
3. Adenoma sebaceum

69. a. True b. True c. True d. False e. True

Also drug abuse, e.g., heroin addicts, infected venous catheter or pacemaker wire, immunodeficiency, CHD, arterio venous catheter.

70.	a. True	b. True	c. False	d. True	e. True
71.	a. True	b. True	c. True	d. False	e. True
72.	a. False	b. True	c. False	d. False	e. False

Turner's syndrome is associated with co-arctation of aorta, bicuspid aortic valve, dissection aorta, etc.

73. a. True   b. True c. True   d. True   e. False

74. a. False   b. True   c. False   d. False e. True

75. a. True   b. True   c. True   d. True   e. False

76. a. False b. False c. True   d. True   e. True

Others e.g. pernicious anaemia, in pregnancy, high risk of miscarriage, stillbirth, and low birth weight.

77. a. True b. True c. True d. False e. True

Also broad chest, short status dissection aorta, aortic valve stenosis, hearing loss, horseshoe kidney, co-arctation of oarta, and primary amenorrhoea.

78. a. True   b. True c. True   d. True e. False

79. a. True b. True c. True d. True e. False

80. a. True   b. True   c. True   d. True   e. False

81. a. True   b. True c. True   d. False e. False

82. a. False   b. False c. False   d. True   e. True

Hampton's hump sign is wedge-shaped density at periphery of lung described as a sign of pulmonary embolism. Knuckle sign is dilation pulmonary artery with abrupt tapering seen in occlusive disease like pulmonary embolism. Dense hilum sign appearance of hilum which is neither enlarged nor calcified implying superimposed lung density. Comet tail sign represent lung focal area of collapsed lung adjacent to pleural thickening with distortion of blood vessels in rounded atelectasis. Air crescent sign classically seen in aspirgilloma.

83. a. True   b. True   c. True d. True   e. False

Other causes of vascular calcifications: aneurysm; arteriosclerosis; haemangioma, arteriovenous malformation; hyperparathyroidism, primary or secondary; Monckeberg's sclerosis (medial sclerosis); phleboliths (e.g.,

normal, varicose veins, haemangioma, Maffucci's syndrome, postradiation); premature sclerosis:
- a) Familial hyperlipemia.
- b) Generalised arterial calcification of infancy.
- c) Progeria.
- d) Secodary hyperlipemia:
  1. Cushing's syndrome.
  2. Diabetes mellitus.
  3. Glycogen storage disease.
  4. Hypothyroidism.
  5. Lipodystrophy.
  6. Nephrotic syndrome.
  7. Renal homotransplantation.
- e) Werner's syndrome.

Buerger's disease; burn, frostbite; calcified thrombus (e.g., vena cava, portal vein, arterial); gout, hyperuricemia; homocystinuria; hydramnios in infants; Hypervitaminosis D; hypoparathyroidism; idiopathic hypercalcemia; imoblization syndrome; mucoviscidosis; pseudoxanthoma elasticum; Raynaud's disease; sarcoidosis; Tkayasu's arteritis.

84. a. True   b. True   c. True   d. True   e. False

DiGeorge syndrome is congenital condition characteristic signs and symptoms may include birth defects such as congenital heart disease, defect in the palate, learning disabilities, mild differences in facial features, recurrent infections, hypoplastic thymus, hypocalcemia due to malfunctioning parathyroid glands, thrombocytopenia, etc.

85. a. True   b. True   c. True   d. False   e. True

86. a. False   b. True   c. True   d. True   e. True

87. a. True   b. False   c. True   d. True   e. True

1. The following are true in Stein-Leventhal syndrome (Polycystic ovary syndrome):
   a) Menopause age.
   b) Associated with thyroid tumour.
   c) Cystic acne.
   d) Endometrial cancer is common.
   e) Bilateral enlarged polycystic ovaries.
2. Hydronephrosis in pregnancy:
   a) Usually occur in the 1st and 2nd trimester.
   b) Left kidney commonly affected.
   c) Associated with staghorn calculi.
   d) Asymptomatic.
   e) Resolution after delivery.

3. In Wilm's tumour the following are true:
   a) May be bilateral.
   b) Commonly metastases to the bone.
   c) Commonest age to presentation is before 3 years.
   d) Commonest abdominal tumour in children.
   e) Associated with hemihypertrophy.

4. The following are true in Benign Prostate Hypertrophy:
   a) Prostate specific antigens (PSA) typically elevated.
   b) Alpha blockers are the most common choice for initial therapy.
   c) Transrectal ultrasonogrphy is contraindicated in advance cases.
   d) The maximum volume of prostate by ultrasound about 30 cc.
   e) Bladder calculi are recognised complication.

5. In duplex kidney:
   a) Males are more affected than females.
   b) Commoner on the left than the right.
   c) Associated with multiple renal arteries.
   d) Obstruction more commonly involves the upper moiety.
   e) Reflux is more common into the lower moiety.

6. The following conditions demonstrate segmental cortical defects on enhanced CT:
   a) Renal artery branch stenosis.
   b) Renal tuberculosis.
   c) Transitional cell carcinoma.
   d) Glomerular nephritis.
   e) Stag horn calculus.

7. The following in tailgut cyst are true:
   a) About half of presacral tumours are congenital lesion.
   b) Commonly male child.
   c) It can be asymptomatic.
   d) MRI is the imaging modality to confirm the diagnosis.
   e) It may be multiple.

8. When using ultrasound in obstetric:
   a) Twins can be diagnosed at 15 weeks.
   b) Anterior placenta previa can be diagnosed with confidence at 25 weeks.
   c) Ultrasound is more accurate than x-ray from 36 weeks until term.
   d) An empty bladder, essential for pelvic examination.
   e) More accurate from 20–32 weeks.

9. Causes of primary amenorrhea may be:
   a) Stein- Leventhial syndrome.
   b) Anorexia nervosa.
   c) Chronic renal failure.
   d) Endometriosis.
   e) Asherman syndrome.

10. The following are true in perinephric abscess:
    a) Lateral displacement of duodeno-jejunal flexure.
    b) Loss of psoas outline.

c) Reduced renal substances.
   d) Loss of peritoneal fat line.
   e) Lack of movement of respiration.

11. Renal tuberculosis may cause:
    a) Parenchymal calcification.
    b) Strictures usually Pelviureteric junction obstruction (PUJ).
    c) A dilated floppy bladder.
    d) Vesical lesion resembling a carcinoma.
    e) Autonephractomy.

12. Ultrasound of female:
    a) It is normal to have an endometrial thickness of 5 mm in the 24th day of the cycle.
    b) It is normal to have an endometrial thickness of 5 mm in the 19th day of the cycle.
    c) There is a narrow zone of hydroechogenicity under the endometrial echo during proliferative phase.
    d) The endometrial echogenicity increases during the secretory phase.
    e) In postmenopausal age group, the endometrial thickness reduces even if having hormonal replacement therapy.

13. In neonatal adrenal haemorrhage:
    a) Diabetic mother.
    b) Bilateral 90% of cases.
    c) Associated with birth trauma.
    d) Newborns maybe presented with anaemia, jaundice, or adrenal insufficiency.
    e) Occurs more often on the left side.

14. The indication of scrotal ultrasound are:
    a) Inguinal hernia.
    b) Hypogonadism.
    c) Cryptorchism.
    d) Prostatic mass.
    e) Urethral valve.

15. Content of anterior pararenal space:
    a) Pancreas.
    b) Ascending colon.

c)   Duodenum.
   d)   Proximal small bowel loop.
   e)   Adrenal glands.

16. The following are true in testicular neoplasm:
    a)   Most common malignancy in age group 15–35 years.
    b)   Commonly in African origin.
    c)   95% are germ cell tumours.
    d)   95% can be detected by ultrasound.
    e)   Normal size test and normal echotexture is common.

17. In acute pyelonephritis:
    a)   Focal swelling and decreased perfusion of affected parenchyma.
    b)   Commonly associated with vesicoureteral reflux.
    c)   Commonly bilateral.
    d)   Wedge-shaped peripheral low density area on CT scan.
    e)   Poor corticomedullary differentiation on ultrasound.

18. The following statements are true:
    a)   Idiopathc Hypercalcemia (William's syndrome) associated with peculiar elfin like facies.
    b)   25% of mongolism has 11 rib pairs.
    c)   Enlarged azygous vein seen in Scimitar syndrome.
    d)   Pelvic lipomatosis can cause a pear-shaped bladder.
    e)   There is association between chronic glomerulonephritis and pulmonary calcification.

19. Dense persistence nephrogram on CT scan seen in:
    a)   Hypertension.
    b)   Renal failure.
    c)   Bilateral renal vein thrombosis.
    d)   Ischemia.
    e)   Multiple myeloma.

20. In vesicoureteral reflux seen:
    a)   Urethral valve.
    b)   Constipation.
    c)   Hirschsprung's disease.
    d)   Prune belly syndrome.
    e)   Colonic diverticulum.

21. In ureterocele:
    a) Simple ureterocele located in the trigone of the bladder.
    b) Ectopic ureterocele may insert into vagina.
    c) Ectopic type is less common than the simple type.
    d) VCUG is best test to assess dynamic nature of the ureterocele.
    e) MRI is useful to delineate associated gynecologic abnormalities seen in 50% of women with duplication.

22. Renal vein thrombosis occurring in children is:
    a) Most common in the 1st year of life.
    b) Usually related to gastroenteritis.
    c) Associated with enlarged kidney.
    d) Not associated with Hematuria.
    e) Not associated with glucosuria.

23. The following are true of the posterior urethral valves:
    a) Associated with prune belly system.
    b) Associated with vesico-ureteric reflux.
    c) Occur proximal to the verumontanum.
    d) Are better seen on the micturating cysto-urethrography than on cystoscopy.
    e) Incidence is the same in both males and females.

24. The following are features of posterior urethra valves:
    a) Ascites may be a presenting feature.
    b) Respiratory difficulty.
    c) Dilated ureters.
    d) Initial presentation may occur after 20 years of age.
    e) They may be adequately diagnosed by retrograde ureterography.

25. In hydrops fetalis on plain x-ray there may be:
    a) Loss of the fetal line.
    b) An abnormal position of the fetus.
    c) Calcification in the fetal abdomen.
    d) An abnormal position of fetal arm and legs.
    e) No radiological abnormality.

26. The following are features of prune belly syndrome:
    a) Imperforate anus.
    b) Hydronephrosis.
    c) Intestinal malrotation.

d) Macrocephaly.
e) Bilateral undescended testes.

27. In schistosomiasis:
    a) Presented with heamaturia and albuminuria.
    b) Sqaumous cell carcinoma of the bladder is common.
    c) May affected the GI tract and causes portal hypertension.
    d) Ureteritis cystic is a remote possibility.
    e) Scrotal abscess is common.

28. In fetal ascites is:
    a) Seen on ultrasound in 5–10% of normal fetuses.
    b) Associated with urinary tract obstruction.
    c) Associated with 'prune belly' syndrome.
    d) Associated with rhesus incompatibility.
    e) Associated with duodenal atresia.

29. Intra abdominal calcifications in fetus seen in:
    a) Cytomegalovirus.
    b) Teratoma.
    c) Wilm's tumour.
    d) Metastatic neuroblastoma.
    e) Hepatoplastoma.

30. Which x-ray changes may suggest intra-uterine death of fetus:
    a) Spalding's sign.
    b) Westermark's sign.
    c) Deuel's halo sign.
    d) Gas in the fetal vessels.
    e) The silhouette sign.

31. Bilateral large kidneys in adult seen in:
    a) Acromegaly.
    b) Advance (old) renal cortical necrosis.
    c) Sarcoidosis.
    d) Beer-drinker's kidney.
    e) Myelomatosis.

32. Ultrasound examination may produce characteristics results in:
    a) Acute small bowel obstruction.
    b) Pulmonary metastases.

c) Mitral stenosis.
d) Hydatidiform mole.
e) Renal cyst.

33. Bilateral large kidney in the infant may be due to:
    a) Diabetic mother.
    b) Glycogen storage disease.
    c) Thalassemia.
    d) Tuberous sclerosis.
    e) Laurence-Moon-Biedl syndrome.

34. Avascular renal mass on angiogram can be due to:
    a) Hematoma.
    b) Neuroblastoma.
    c) Fibroma.
    d) Angiofibrolipoma.
    e) Xanthogranulomatous pyelonephritis.

35. In urethral diverticulum:
    a) Common in women about 40 years of age.
    b) Hematuria and/or recurrent urinary tract infections are common clinical findings.
    c) Voiding cystourethrography (VCUG) should be avoided.
    d) Endorectal ultrasound is contraindicated.
    e) Carcinoma can develop within a diverticulum.

36. The following are associated with the administration of drugs during pregnancy:
    a) Hip dysplasia.
    b) Phocomelia.
    c) Marfan's.
    d) Hypoplasia of the radius.
    e) Pseudoarthrosis.

37. A pear-shaped bladder may be seen in:
    a) Inferior vena cava obstruction.
    b) Pelvic lipomatosis.
    c) Prostate tumour.
    d) Neurogenic bladder.
    e) Hodgkin's disease.

38. With uterine fibroids following can happen:
    a) Infertility.
    b) Malignancy.
    c) Postpartum haemorrhage.
    d) Hydatidiform mole.
    e) Ovarian neoplasm.

39. Bladder diverticula the following are true:
    a) Hutch diverticula are congenital common in males and is solitary usually.
    b) It can be longer than the bladder itself.
    c) Voiding cystogram is contra indicating.
    d) Stone formation within the diverticula is likely present.
    e) Epithelial dysplasia is recognised complication.

40. Diverticulosis of fallopian tube:
    a) Increase incidence of ectopic pregnancy.
    b) Fistula in the colon may develop.
    c) Associated with previous tuberculus infection.
    d) Almost always multiple.
    e) Commonly in white > black.

41. Congenital dislocation of the hip is associated with:
    a) Breech.
    b) Commoner in males.
    c) Family history.
    d) Spina bifida.
    e) Diabetic mother.

42. In retro peritoneal fibrosis :
    a) Backache.
    b) Do not respond to steroids.
    c) Associated with lymphatic obstruction at that level.
    d) Complication of analgesic abuse.
    e) Retrograde pyelogram is contraindicated.

43. Renal cell carcinoma may be associated with:
    a) Cushing syndrome.
    b) Polycythemia.
    c) Hypercalcemia.

d) Thrombophlebitis (IVC thrombosis).
e) Hypertension.

44. In retrocaval ureter:
   a) Ascending urethrogram is contraindicating.
   b) Commonly old females.
   c) The right ureter course behind the inferior vena cava.
   d) Staghorn calculi is a common complication.
   e) Associated with horseshoe kidney.

45. Causes of interarenal artery aneurysm on angiogram are:
   a) Polyarteritis nodosa.
   b) Wegner's granuloma.
   c) Horseshoe kidney.
   d) Renal cell carcinoma.
   e) Hypoplastic kidney.

46. In medullary sponge kidney the following are true:
   a) Renal function impaired.
   b) The affected kidney is normal in size.
   c) Associated with hepatic fibrosis.
   d) Increased serum calcium.
   e) There is usually vesico ureteric reflux.

47. The following are true in angiomyolipoma:
   a) It may be hepatic.
   b) Associated with neurofibromatosis.
   c) Haemorrhagic shock due to massive interperitonium bleeding may happen.
   d) May be the only evidence of tuberous sclerosis.
   e) Always bilateral.

48. Pelvic congestion syndrome is true:
   a) Associated with ectopic pregnancy.
   b) Associated with uretro-dermoid cyst.
   c) Associated with cystic ovaries.
   d) Associated with retroperitoneal fibrosis.
   e) Associated with pelvic lipomatosis.

49. In bladder cancer:
    a) Classic clinical presentation painful hematuria.
    b) Smoking is a risk factor.
    c) It can be multicentric.
    d) Associated with schistosoma haemotubium-infected patients.
    e) It gives a filling defect on cystography.

50. Following are true in osteitis condensans ilii:
    a) Usually painless and symmetrical.
    b) Associated with ankylosing spondylitis.
    c) Morning stiffness and polyarthralgia.
    d) Maybe osteolytic.
    e) May spontaneously resolve.

51. In kidneys:
    a) The kidneys measures 11–15 cm.
    b) The right kidney is longer than the left by 1.5 cm.
    c) The upper pole of the kidneys lies medially and anteriorly.
    d) The columns of Bertin separate the medulla into pyramids.
    e) The renal papilla is a component of the pyramid.

52. Abdominal lymph nodes, the following are true:
    a) Presence of enlarged left gastric nodes indicate grave prognosis in esophageal cancers.
    b) There are more than 100 lymph glands in the mesentery.
    c) There are predominantly four group of mesenteric lymph nodes.
    d) Epicolic nodes are close to the large bowel wall.
    e) Perirectal nodes are in the wall of the rectum.

53. In uterus:
    a) Cervical canal usually measures 2 cm.
    b) Cervical canal is spindles shaped.
    c) Normal uterus measures up to 35 mm and has higher vertical than coronal dimension.
    d) Fallopian tubes can measure 10 cm or more.
    e) Fallopian tubes have columner epithelium.

54. Ultrasound of ectopic pregnancy may be true:
    a) 25% have detectable heart beat.
    b) Fluid in pouch of Douglas excludes the diagnosis.
    c) Absence of fluid in the pouch of Douglas excludes the diagnosis.

d) GIFT increased the incidence of coexistent intrauterine foetus and ectopic.
e) 95% of ectopic pregnancy have positive pregnancy test.

55. Associations of medullary sponge kidney:
    a) Fanconi's syndrome (pancytopenia-dymelia syndrome).
    b) Beckwith-Wiedemann syndrome.
    c) Congenital hypertrophic pyloric stenosis.
    d) Parathyroid adenoma.
    e) Marfan's syndrome.

56. Micturating cystourethrography (MCU):
    a) Cystography can differentiate mechanical and neurogenic cause of dysfunction.
    b) Stress incontinence is the most common indication of cystography.
    c) The bladder has more height than width in woman.
    d) Oblique views are avoided during micturition.
    e) Dysuria following MCU suggests infection.

57. In renal infarction:
    a) Seen in sickle cell disease.
    b) Seen in polyarteritis nodosa.
    c) Seen in sub acute bacterial endocarditis.
    d) Parenchymal renal infarction are best demonstrated on CT scan.
    e) Hydronephrosis.

58. In renal failure tubular rather than glomerular damage predominates:
    a) Myelomatosis.
    b) Analgesic nephropathy.
    c) Diabetes mellitus.
    d) Amyloid.
    e) Crush syndrome.

59. Erythrocytemia occurs in:
    a) Renal cell carcinoma.
    b) Renal adenoma.
    c) Haemangiopercytoma.
    d) Hepatoma.
    e) Haemangioma.

60. In renal tumour:
    a) Partial nephrectomy is precluded if adrenal gland is involved.
    b) Incidence of metastasis is higher by 50% in those with loco-reginal lymph nodes.
    c) Renal vein extension occurs in only 1% of RCC at presentation.
    d) IVC extension occurs in 5–10% of tumours at presentation.
    e) Embolic thrombus involves supra hepatic portion of IVC in 40% of cases.

61. The following are true in benign Adrenal Adenoma:
    a) On non-enhanced CT scan, it looks as small size less than 3 cm in diameter, smooth round well-defined contour, attenuation less than 10 H.
    b) Calcification is common on CT scan.
    c) It arises from the cortex of the gland.
    d) It can be an incidental finding on CT scan examination in non-symptomatic patient.
    e) It is difficult to distinguish from benign adrenal cyst on NECT.

62. The following are true in carcinoid tumours adenoma:
    a) Low grade malignancies about 90% metastasize.
    b) Female to male ratio of 10:1.
    c) Black to white ratio of 5:1.
    d) The salivary gland type cylindromas is more common than mucoepidermoid type.
    e) Very few carcinoids of the lung give rise to carcinoid syndrome.

63. In testicular torsion (acute scrotum):
    a) Sonography and nuclear imaging studies both demonstrate decreased or absent perfusion of the testes.
    b) Men over 40 most often affected.
    c) Left side affected more often than right.
    d) It is considered as surgical emergency.
    e) Shrunken and/or calcified testicle on CT or MRI scans indicating missed torsion.

64. The following statements are true in regard to polycalycosis (megacalyces syndrome):
    a) It is characterised by non-obstructive enlargement of the minor calyces.
    b) It has a recognised association with megaureter.

c) The affected kidney is usually small.
d) Calculus formation is a recognised complication.
e) It is usually diagnosed as an incidental finding on intravenous urography.

65. In Goodpasture's syndrome:
    a) Pulmonary haemorrhage.
    b) Glomerulonephrosis.
    c) It is a disease of children.
    d) May have pulmonary hypertension.
    e) May have hilar adenopathy.

66. A flank mass and an ipsilateral non-functioning kidney should suggest:
    a) Wilm's tumour.
    b) Multicystic kidney.
    c) Pelvi-ureteric obstruction.
    d) Retro-caval ureter.
    e) Polycystic kidney.

67. In adult polycystic kidney:
    a) Associated with pancreatic cyst.
    b) Azotemia.
    c) Cyst may calcified.
    d) Clear renal contour.
    e) Berry aneurysm.

68. In pheochromocytoma:
    a) 100% adrenal medulla.
    b) Associated with tuberous sclerosis.
    c) IV injection of iodinated contrast material may precipitate hypertensive crisis in patients not on alpha-adrenergic block.
    d) 10% malignant.
    e) Extremely hyperintense to liver on T2W1.

69. In unilateral small kidney:
    a) Obstructive uropathy.
    b) Renal artery stenosis.
    c) Fibromuscular hyperplasia.
    d) Kimmelestial-Wilson disease.
    e) Chronic glomerulonephritis.

70. In ascending urethrography:
    a) Spasm is reduced by avoiding warm contrast medium.
    b) Balloon catheter should be inflated in the membranous urethra to retain the catheter.
    c) The best procedure for demonstrating prostatic urethra.
    d) 30 degrees oblique are taken on both side.
    e) Urethral fistula is best seen in injection phase.

71. Causes of chyluria:
    a) Filariasis.
    b) Thoracic aortic aneurysm.
    c) Pelvic lipomatosis.
    d) Pregnancy.
    e) Schistosomiasis.

72. Bladder rupture the following are true:
    a) Extraperitoneal bladder rupture is the most common type.
    b) Blunt trauma in an adult can result in interperitoneal rupture only if the bladder is fully distended.
    c) Voiding cystourethrography (VCUG) is contraindicating in suspected intraperitoneal bladder rupture.
    d) Bladder within a bladder seen on ultrasound.
    e) Extraperitoneal bladder rupture treated conservatively in most of the cases.

73. In pancreatic disease – panniculitis syndrome (PPP):
    a) Approximately up to 3% of patients with pancreatic disease also present themselves with panniculitis and/or arthritis.
    b) Panniculitis in the PPP syndrome typically affecting the lower limb.
    c) Typical radiological findings are multiple osteolytic lesions.
    d) Typical patient is a middle-aged man with history of heavy alcoholic abuse.
    e) Isotope scan is the most sensitive imaging method for detecting PPP.

74. MRI in renal tumours:
    a) Tumours thrombosis is seen as high signal lesion in spin echo images.
    b) MRI has accuracy in 100% for vena caval involvement.

c) MRI has superior accuracy than CT in assessment of lymph nodal involvement.
d) Contrast enhanced spiral CT scan is the best method of staging renal cell carcinoma.
e) MRI is useful for detection of small renal tumours.

75. Erythrocytemia occurs in:
    a) Renal cell carcinoma.
    b) Renal adenoma.
    c) Hemangiopericytoma.
    d) Hepatoma.
    e) Haemangioma.

76. The following associated with abnormal development of limbs in the fetus:
    a) Star-gazing fetus.
    b) Amelia.
    c) Hemimelia.
    d) Phocomelia.
    e) Symmelia.

77. In scar endomteriosis:
    a) Occurring in a caesarean section scar.
    b) MRI is the most sensitive imaging modality.
    c) Usually multiple.
    d) Cystic changes are usual.
    e) Usually intermittent pain associated with the patient's menstrual cycle.

78. Ultrasound is of value in the diagnosis of:
    a) Renal cyst.
    b) Staghorn calculus.
    c) Chronic pyelonephritis.
    d) Papillary necrosis.
    e) Hydronephrosis.

79. The following are features of Conn's syndrome:
    a) Polyuria.
    b) Hypertension.
    c) Hypokalemia.

d) Seizures.
e) Liver cirrhosis.

80. In skene gland cyst:
    a) Normally has a connection with the urethra.
    b) It has no connection with the vagina.
    c) Sometime called female prostate.
    d) Normal location in the posterior introitus.
    e) Containing clear fluid.

81. In oligohydramnios seen:
    a) Post dates.
    b) Diabetes.
    c) Renal abnormalities.
    d) Premature rupture of membrane.
    e) Oesophageal atresia.

82. In turner's syndrome:
    a) Abnormal kidneys.
    b) Low set ear.
    c) Long fingers and toes.
    d) Early fused epiphysis.
    e) Prenatal ultrasound can show cardiac abnormalities.

83. Bear paw sign (dilated renal calyces with normal renal pelvis) seen in:
    a) Horseshoe kidney.
    b) Calculus diseases.
    c) Xanthogranulomatosis.
    d) Pyelonephritis.
    e) Glomerulonephritis.

84. Which of the following is not contraindication to pregnancy:
    a) Large secundum atrial septal defect with left to right shunt.
    b) Marfan syndrome with dilated aorta.
    c) Sever obstructive valvular lesions.
    d) Sever pulmonary hypertension.
    e) Scimitar syndrome.

85. Prevention of contrast nephropathy in risky patients:
    a) Non-ionic low osmolar contrast agents are preferred.
    b) Patient should be hydrated.

c) The amount of contrast media used should be limited.
d) Skin test indicated prior to the injection.
e) No contrast should be given in patients with renal dysfunction.

86. Weight gain in pregnancy depends on:
    a) Pre-pregnancy weight.
    b) Maternal age.
    c) Smoking.
    d) Ethnicity.
    e) Alcoholic mother.

87. In ureteritis cystica:
    a) Perforation is common.
    b) Associated with urenoma.
    c) Multiple 2–5 mm filling defects within the ureter.
    d) Premalignant.
    e) Can involve the renal pelvis as well as the ureters.

88. The abdominal aorta in spina bifida cystica:
    a) The position of the bifurcation is high to the level of the renal arteries.
    b) Aorta is small in calibre.
    c) Horseshoe kidney is an association.
    d) Urethral valve is common association.
    e) Associated with kyphosis.

89. Loss of axillary hair occurs in:
    a) Addison's disease.
    b) Cushing's syndrome.
    c) Hypopitruitism.
    d) Turner's syndrome.
    e) Polycystic ovaries.

90. Horseshoe kidney associated with:
    a) Hypospadias.
    b) Polysplenia.
    c) Retrocaval ureter.
    d) Imporforated anus.
    e) Meckel diverticulum.

91. Endocrinal causes of generalised osteoporosis occurs in:
    a) Addison's disease.
    b) Testicular eunuchoidism.
    c) Basophilic adenoma.
    d) Oat cell carcinoma.
    e) Cretinism.

92. The following are features of Conn's syndrome:
    a) Hypernatremia.
    b) Hypertension.
    c) Hypokalemia.
    d) Hypothyroidism.
    e) Skin pigmentation.

93. In Diverticulosis of the fallopian tube:
    a) There is an increase incidence of ectopic pregnancy.
    b) Fistula into colon may develop.
    c) Is associated with previous tuberculosis infection.
    d) Common in West Indian.
    e) Associated with twin pregnancy.

94. The presence of hydrominos should suggest:
    a) Anencephaly.
    b) Oesophageal atresia.
    c) Duodenal atresi.
    d) Renal anomalies.
    e) Placenta previa.

95. The following are true in perinephric abscess:
    a) Lateral displacement of duodeno-jejunal flexure.
    b) Loss of psoas outline.
    c) Reduced renal substances.
    d) Loss of retroperitoneal fat line.
    e) Lack of movement of respiration.

96. In inferior vena cava thrombosis:
    a) Medial deviation of ureters.
    b) Increased pre sacral space.
    c) Splenomegaly.
    d) Bilateral renal enlargement.
    e) Can be diagnosed by C.T. Scan.

97. Types of female pelvic inlets are true:
    a) Gynaecoid type has optimum round pelvic brim.
    b) Android type has a triangular brim shape.
    c) Anthropoid type has an inlet of a long oval shape and the conjugate is greater than the transverse.
    d) Robert pelvis is asymmetrical deformity of the inlet.
    e) Platypelloid has a broad or flat at the inlet, the transverse diameter being well in excess of the conjugate.

98. In epidermoid cyst of the testicle:
    a) The lesion occurs in the 2st decade of life
    b) Ultrasound is the study of choice will show a round well demarcated intratesticular mass with internal hetrogenecity(onion skin) appearance
    c) Hypervascular on color imaging
    d) Absence of enhancement with contrast on MRI imaging
    e) Asymptomatic usually.

99. Duodenal obstruction in an infant seen in:
    a) Cholodochal cyst.
    b) Annular pancreas.
    c) Duplication of duodenum.
    d) Superior mesenteric artery syndrome.
    e) Diabetic mother.

100. In hydrops fetalis:
    a) Oligohydramnios is a feature.
    b) Fetal ascites can be seen on ultrasound.
    c) Rhesus incompatibility exists between mother and fetus.
    d) There is neonatal anaemia.
    e) There is increased placental width on ultrasound.

101. Non-visceral abdominal calcification:
    a) Armillifer armillatus infestation.
    b) Meconium peritonitis.
    c) Histocytosis.
    d) Tuberculus peritonitis.
    e) Dermoid cyst.

1. a. False   b. False   c. True   d. True   e. True

Stein-Leventhal Syndrome (Polycystic Ovary Syndrome)
Pearly white ovaries with multiple cysts. Occurs 2nd decade incidence 2.5% of all women.
Associated with Cushing syndrome, basophilic pituitary adenoma, post pill amenorrhea, virilizing ovarian, adrenal tumour. Reduced infertility/sterility, generalised hirtuism, obesity, bilaterally enlarged ovaries, endometrial cancer < 40 years.

2. a. False   b. False   c. False   d. True   e. True

Hydronephrosis in pregnancy is about 80–90% by the 3rd trimester, affected the right side is about 80–90%. Likely cause is hormonal in response to progesterone the smooth muscle of the ureter relaxed and dilated only to the pelvic brim. It is usually asymptomatic; however pain mimicking renal colic may occur. Resolution is within a few weeks to 6 months after delivery.

3. a. True   b. False   c. True   d. True   e. True

Wilm's tumour (nephroblastoma) is a cancer of the kidney in children: 50% < 2 years, bilateral 5% associated with hemihypertrophy.

Calcification < 15%; vascular invasion in < 10%; metastases to the lung and liver 50%.

4. a. False   b. True   c. False   d. True   e. True

Benign Prostatic Hyperplasia also called benign enlargement of the prostate, adenofibromyomatous hyperplasia, and benign prostatic hyperatrophy.

When sufficiently large, the nodules compress the urethral canal to cause partial or sometimes virtually complete, obstruction of the urethra. BPH does not lead to cancer or increase the risk of cancer.

Rectal examination may reveal a markedly enlarged prostate usually affecting the middle lobe. Transrectal ultrasonography can provide early detection. Prostate Specific Antigen (PSA) level in the blood is not affected.

Some signs of BPH include weak urinary stream, prolonged emptying of the bladder, abdominal straining—post urination dribble, nocturia, bladder pain, Dysuria, problem in ejaculation. Complication includes urinary bladder calculi and diverticula, hydronephrosis, urine retention, recurrent gross haematuria.

5. a. False   b. True   c. True   d. True   e. True

Duplication of the renal pelvis and ureter, the result of abnormal division of the ureteric bud is a common anomaly. Complete duplication involves the renal pelvis and whole length of the ureter so that each division of the pelvis is drained by its own ureter opening separately into the bladder. The ureter cross in the abdomen or pelvis so that the ureter draining the upper renal segment always open below and medial to the ureteric orifice for the lower segment.

6. a. True   b. True   c. False   d. False   e. False

Lobulation of the kidney in the normal kidney persistence of focal lobulation may simulate a tumour and the frequent occurrence of bulge on the normal left kidney. Hypertrophy of the normal renal tissue adjacent to the scars of chronic pyelonephritis or renal infarcts produces a localised thickening of the renal substance with bulge on the renal surface but the true nature of these lesions can be seen by enhanced CT scan. Fibrolipomatosis of the renal hilum my occasionally cause elongation of the calyses and simulate a central or hilar renal mass. These cases show areas of increased activity while tumours and cyst give area of decreased activity.

7. a. True   b. False   c. True   d. True   e. True

Tailgut cyst (TGC) or retrorectal cystic hematoma is a rare developmental lesion thought to arise from embryonic post anal gut. It is a uniocular mass situated in the retrorectal space that does not communicate with the rectal lumen. More common in middle-aged women and is often incidentally discovered. Patients may present with symptoms resulting from local mass effect (constipation, rectal fullness, lower abdominal pain, Dysuria, urinary frequency, or additional complication). Palpable pararectal mass may be appreciated at digital rectal examination. Possible complications include infection, fistulisation, and bleeding, few cases of malignant degeneration have been documented.

Surgical excision is mandatory to confirm the diagnosis. MRI is the imaging modality. Uncomplicated TGC shows thin unenhancing or slightly enhancing wall cyst content has signal intensity on T1W images indicates the presence of mucinous proteic, or haemorrhagic material. Multiple cyst and the septa can be present.

8. a. True   b. False   c. True   d. False   e. True

Placenta
Measurement of final placenta: diameter – 15–20 cm; weight – 600 gram; thickness – < 4 cm.
Ultrasound feature: hypoechoic relative to adjacent myometrium; draining veins can be seen in the basal plate; calcifications are physiologic and have no clinical significance; normal hypoechoic or anechoic foci in placenta may present fibrin, thrombus, material-like cysts.

It's called placenta previa when covers the internal cervical os.

Placenta accrete there is a loss of the normal placenta/myometrium border. The risk of placenta accrete is higher in patient with prior C-section.

9. a. True   b. True   c. True   d. False   e. False

Primary amenorrhea, mean no menarche in young age, adrenarche by 14 years of age. Due to automatic anomalies Mullerian (uterovaginal) anomalies or congenital disorders of sexual differentiation. Ovarian failure, hypothalamic or pituitary causes, systemic, psychiatric illness and others including irradiation chemotherapy, autoimmune oophoritis, and other syndrome, e.g., turner, polycystic ovary syndrome (may cause secondary type).

10. a. False   b. True   c. True   d. True   e. True

Perinephric Abscess
Usual causes:
1. Extraurinary infection with direct or haematogenous spread.
    a. Deep infection (e.g., Osteomyelitis, laryngitis, tonsillitis, perforated ulcer, diverticulitis, pancreatitis).
    b. Superficial infection (e.g., carbuncle, wound infection).
2. Instrumentation (e.g., removal of Ureteral calculus).
3. Obstructive uropathy.
4. Direct trauma to kidney and ureter.
5. Urinary tract infection (esp. in diabetic women).

11. a. True   b. False   c. False   d. True   e. True

Renal Tuberculosis
Tubercle bacilli reach the kidney via the blood stream and are arrested in a glomerulus with development of the tubercles in the renal cortex. The tubercles are nearly always bilateral and the majority heal. Calcification may occur and the renal outline interrupted probably due to abscesses formation, fibrosis, Ureteral obstruction, and atrophy. Non-functioning kidney with calcification (autonephractomy) is a late stage.

12. a. True   b. False   c. True   d. True   e. True

During menstrual and proliferative phase, the endometrial thickness is up to 4mm, slightly echogenic with a thin hypoechoic myometrium seen underneath.

In secretory phase, the endometrium is more echogenic and can be up to 8mm.

In postmenopausal age, the endometrium thins, unless the patient is on HRT.

13. a. False   b. False   c. True   d. True   e. False

14. a. True   b. True   c. True   d. False   e. False

15. a. True   b. True   c. True   d. False   e. False

The anterior pararenal space is between the anterior layer of gerotus fascia and peritoneum. Descending colon is another content.

16. a. True   b. False   c. True   d. True   e. False

17. a. True   b. True   c. False   d. True   e. True

18. a. True   b. True   c. False   d. True   e. True

19. a. False   b. True   c. True   d. True   e. True

20. a. True   b. True   c. True   d. True   e. False

21. a. True   b. True   c. False   d. True   e. True

22. a. True   b. True   c. True   d. True   e. False

23. a. True   b. True   c. True   d. True   e. False

24. a. False   b. True   c. True   d. True   e. False

25. a. True   b. True   c. True   d. True   e. False

26. a. True   b. True   c. True   d. False   e. True

27. a. True   b. True   c. True   d. False   e. False

28. a. False   b. True   c. True   True   e. False

29. a. True   b. True   c. False   d. True   e. True

30. a. True   b. False   c. True   d. True   e. False

31. a. True   b. False   c. True   d. True   e. True

32. a. False   b. False   c. True   d. True   e. True

33. a. True   b. True   c. False   d. True   e. False

34. a. True   b. False   c. True   d. False   e. True

35. a. True   b. True   c. False   d. False   e. True

Urethral Diverticulum
- Early symptoms – dysuria, frequency, post-micturation dribbling.
- Later symptoms – pelvic pain, dyspareunia.

Imaging Findings
- Voiding cystourethrography (VCUG) is still probably the imaging study of first choice, about 65% accurate.
- Sometimes, diverticulum fills during voiding phase and is best visualised on post-void film.
- Diverticulum will appear as a contrast-containing structure attached to the urethra.
- Positive-pressure urethrography (double balloon catheter studies) generally reserved for cases where findings on VCUG are negative but a diverticulum is strongly suspected. Can be performed with balloons inflated in bladder and at external meatus to 'seal urethra' with central portion of catheter filling urethral itself.
- Ultrasound, either abdominal, vaginal, or endorectal, may also demonstrate urethral diverticula.
- MRI has also been used:
    - T1 shows medium signal intensity, usually homogenous.
    - On T2, fluid shows high signal intensity.

Complications:
- In as many as 10% of cases, stones may form within the diverticular sac may be multiple, usually calcium oxalate or calcium phosphate stones.
- May be associated with varying degrees of inflammation (diverticulitis).
- May rupture into space between periurethral connective tissue and the vaginal wall.
- Rarely, carcinoma develops within a diverticulum.

36. a. False   b. True   c. False   d. False   e. False

Phocomelia is absence of the proximal segment of the limb. Seen in woman on Thalidamid drugs during pregnancy.

Amelia means absence of limb. Symmelia is fusion of the limbs in whole, if partly fused called mermaid. Hemimelia is absence of distal part of a limb.

37. a. True   b. True   c. False   d. True   e. True

A deformed shaped urinary bladder occurs in may condition and give different shapes, e.g., pear shape or pine tree shape or hour-glass bladder, vesical diverticulum, neurogenic bladder.

Some cause of pear-shaped urinary bladder, neurogenic bladder, pelvic masses, e.g., enlarged lymph glands or pelvic lipomatosis, or trauma.

38. a. True   b. True   c. True   d. False   e. False

Uterine Fibroids
- Uterine fibroids are leiomyomas, benign tumours of smooth muscle origin.
- Occur in between 20–50% of women > 30 years of age.
- Fibroids may enlarge with elevated oestrogen levels. They enlarge during the first trimester of pregnancy.
- Uterine fibroids diminish in size after menopause.
- More common in blacks than whites (3:1).
- Most are intramural, i.e., middle of myometrium.
- More fibroids are in the fundus and body of the uterus. Others can be subserosal or exophytic, or submucosal and subendometrial (rarely).
- Most women are asymptomatic.
- Symptoms can include menorrhagia (increase duration or flow), frequently from a submucosal fibroid, pain, urinary frequency, or incontinence and infertility.
- Ultrasound is the study of choice.
- Conventional radiography:
    o Soft tissue mass arising in the pelvis but separate from the urinary bladder.
    o Amorphous, flocculent calcifications in the pelvis—may resemble 'popcorn' or may calcify the outer rim of fibroid.
    o Displacement of bowel gas up and out of the pelvis.
- Ultrasound:
    o Echogenic mass if fibrosis prevails.
    o Hypoechoic, solid mass if muscle component is prevalent.
    o Sharp discrete shadows.

- o Anechoic features if central portion of fibroids has degenerated.
- MRI:
  - o Low/intermediate signal intensity of T1 and T2 weighted images.
  - o High central signal intensity on T2 from haemorrhage.
  - o May have hyperintense rim.
  - o With contrast, most are hypointense, about 25% isointense and 10% hyperintense to myometrium.
- CT:
  - o Mass containing mixed densities, low attenuation if necrotic and higher attenuation if calcified or haemorrhagic.
- Infertility from interference with implantation.
- During pregnancy:
  - o Spontaneous abortion.
  - o Intrauterine growth retardation.
  - o Postpartum haemorrhage.

39. a. True   b. True   c. False   d. True   e. True

Bladder Diverticula
- Uncommon.
- May be congenital or acquired:
  - o Congenital (Hutch diverticula) are usually solitary. More common in males.
  - o Acquired arise from obstruction, infection, or iatrogenic. More common than congenital. Multiple and bladder is usually trabeculated.
- Congenital arise from herniation of the mucosa through the musculature of the bladder wall.
- Can become larger than bladder.
- Usually occur lateral and superior to openings of ureters.
- Single diverticula on one or both sides of the bladder may be an incidental finding but multiple diverticula on the same side suggests an underlying condition.
- When symptomatic, may present with urinary tract infection.
- Rarely a cause of bladder outlet obstruction.
- Voiding cystourethrogram (VCUG) is imaging modality most frequently used.
- Ultrasound may demonstrate larger diverticula.

- Narrow-mouthed diverticula will drain slowly and are more prone to stasis and infection than a side-mouthed.
- Congenital forms are most often adjacent to urethral orifice and are more often wide-mouthed.
- Will enlarge as bladder emptied.
- May occur on dome of bladder in bladder outlet obstruction or Eagle Barrett Syndrome (prune belly syndrome).

Differential Diagnosis
- Bladder ears:
    o Protrude through internal inguinal ring.
    o More often seen in children than adults.
    o Seen most often when bladder is maximally distended.
    o Will empty when bladder emptied (diverticula tens to find when bladder emptied).
- Bladder diverticula occur in William's syndrome.
    o Also hypercalcemia and aortic and other stenosis.
- Ehlers-Danlos syndrome, Menkens syndrome also have higher incidence of bladder diverticula.

Complications
- Infection.
- Stones.
  Epithelial dysplasia.
- Vesicoureteral reflux (more common).
- Ureteral obstruction (very rare).
- Bladder outlet obstruction (very rare).

40. a. True   b. True   c. True   d. False   e. False

Diverticulosis of fallopian tube is recognised cause of ectopic pregnancy commonly in West India, Negro, may cause total obstruction of the fallopian tube, may be due to tuberculosis associated with endometriosis and cause colonic fistula.

Easily diagnosed by hystosalphingogram.

41. a. True   b. False   c. True   d. True   e. True

Congenital dislocation of Hip (Hip Dysplasia/ developmental dysplasia/ Congenital Acetabular Dysplasia

- Common in girls.
- Ultrasound is sensitive during first 2 weeks.
- However can be diagnosed up to 4 months.
- Increased amount of soft tissues echoes between femoral head and acetabulum.
- The cartilaginous acetabular labrum interposed between head and acetabulum (inverted labrum).
- Abnormal alpha angle (angle between straight lateral edge of ilium and bony acetabular margin)
- α > 60° is normal in the infant.
- < 50° at birth need to follow up at 4 weeks intervals.
- B angle between straight lateral edge of ilium + fibrocartilaginous acetabulum. B angle < 77°

42. a. True   b. False   c. True   d. True   e. False

Retroperitoneal fibrosis is proliferation of the fibrous tissue in the peritoneal space have been reported following the use of methysergide and other ergot derivatives in the treatment of migraine.

The fibrosis many extend to involve the mediastinum including the coronary arteries.

Blood vessels in the pelvis are also may involve as well as the ureters and bile ducts.

They presented with renal pain, infection, and uraemia.

On full length view intravenous pyelography both the lower ureter are medially displaced.

43. a. False   b. True   c. True   d. True   e. True

Renal Cell Carcinoma
Classically presents with loin pain, fever, haematuria, palpable mass, however the tumour may be silent until for advanced such as metastasis in bones, lung liver, adrenal gland, and the opposite kidney.

May be presented with polycythemia due to the production of erythropoietin by the tumour.

Hypertension and hypercalcemia and anaemia may also be presented. There may be direct extension into the renal veins.

44. a. False   b. False   c. True   d. False   e. True

Retrocaval (Circumcaval) Ureter
- Also known as 'circumcaval ureter'
- Abnormality in embryogenesis of IVC—results from abnormal persistence of right subcardinal vein positioned ventral to ureter in the definitive IVC, developing right ureter courses behind and medial to the IVC.
- Incidence: 0.07%, male to female ratio of 3:1.
- Symptoms of right ureteral obstruction—pain, hematuria.
- Right ureter's course swings medially over pedicle of L3/4 passes behind IVC then exits anteriorly between IVC and aorta returning to its normal position in lower third produces varying degrees of proximal hydroureteronephrosis.
- Can be associated with Turner's syndrome
- The retroperitoneal fibrosis affected the upper ureter, while the lower ureter are affected by lymphadenopathy, iliac artery aneurysm, bladder diverticulum, pelvic lipomatosis, post surgical interventions, or some pelvic masses including hematoma.

45. a. True   b. False   c. False   d. False   e. True

Cause of interarenal artery aneurysm are polyarteritis nodosa, Wegner's granuloma metosis, congenital, atherosclerosis, angiomyolipoma (in tuberous sclerosis) SLE. Drug abuse vasculitus, allergic vasculitis, renal cell carcinoma.

Transplant rejection and neurofibroma.

46. a. False   b. True   c. False   d. False   e. False

Medullary sponge kidney is a congenital disease in which the renal medulla is placed by numerous small cysts producing a sponge-like appearance. The disease may affect the whole or greater part of one or both kidneys. Rarely on papilla may be affected. Calculi may be seen within the cysts. The renal function is unimpaired unless repeated attacks of infection or obstruction. On post IV contrast examination the contrast medium persist in the cysts for some time.

47. a. True   b. True   c. True   d. True   e. False

Angiomyolipomas
- Is benign renal mesenchymal tumour containing, fat, smooth muscle, and thick-walled blood vessels.
- Incidence is up to 3%.
- The vessels do not have a complete elastic layer. Predisposing to aneurysms and haemorrhage. If the tumour is greater than > 4 cm, there is 60% chance of heamorrhage. Angiomyolipoma is sporadic in 80%, and associated with tuberous sclerosis in 20%.
- There is association with Hippel-Lindu syndrome and neurofibromatosis.
- By ultrasound, there is increased echogenicity within a mass.
- On CT, there is variable amount of fat within the lesions and may demonstrate the presence of haemorrhage.
- On MRI, focal fat with high T1W and T2W signal that show signal loss on fat suppression sequences is characteristic.

48. a. False   b. True   c. False   d. False   e. False

Pelvic congestion syndrome is extensive pelvic varices commonly associated with pain and heaviness however may be interfere with movement, posture, and activities that increase abdominal pressure.
Some risk factors are hormonal influence, pelvic surgery, multiple pregnancies can be diagnosed by venography or transvaginal ultrasound and color Doppler commonly. Associated cystic ovaries.

On MRI shows tortuous, enhancing tubular structures near the uterus and ovary on T1-W images varices appear as flow voids.

Gradient-echo MR varices have high signal intensity.

T2W images usually varices appear low in signal intensity.

49. a. False   b. True   c. True   d. True   e. True

Bladder Cancer
- More common in whites than in blacks.
- 3:1 male to female predominance.
- Classical clinical presentation is painless, gross hematuria.
- Risk factors:

- Smoking
- Pelvic irradiation
- Exposure to aniline dyes
- Chemotherapy with clyclosphosphamide
- Most common:
  1. Transitional cell carcinoma
     o Multicentric
     o Tumours may be classified by growth patterns: papillary, sessile or mixed, nodular
  2. Squamous caell carcinoma
     o Worst prognosis, associated with bladder infection by Schistosoma haematobium
  3. Adenocarcinoma (1%)
     o About 5% present with metastatic disease: most often lymph nodes, lung, liver, bone, and central nervous system.

50. a. True   b. False   c. True   d. False   e. True

Osteitis Condensans Ilii
- Benign sclerosis of the iliac side of the sacroiliac joints.
- Bilaterally symmetric, rarely unilateral.
- Usually found in young females who have had several children.
- Related to remodelling of bone following stress across the sacroiliac joint.
- Other theories of etiology are that it is related to a urinary tract infection, or that it may be related to a form of inflammatory arthritis.

Imaging Findings
- Sclerosis is frequently triangular in shape with the base pointing inferiorly not to be confused with a sacroiliitis.
- Sclerosis involves only iliac side of joint in osteitis condensans ilii.
- Outer margin of sclerosis is usually well-defined.
- If in doubt, oblique views of the SI joints will show the joint to be intact and the sclerosis on only iliac side.
- May spontaneously resolve.

51. a. True   b. False   c. False   d. True   e. True

Usually the left kidney is longer than the right by 1.5 cm. The right kidney should be not more than 1.0 cm longer than the left kidney.

The upper poles lie medially and more posteriorly. The renal pyramids have a base, body, apex, and papilla, which projects into the calyx.

52. a. True   b. True   c. False   d. False   e. False

Mesenteric lymph nodes are 3 groups:
1. Mural – near the intestinal wall.
2. Intermediate between the arcades.
3. Juxta arterial – adjacent to superior mesenteric artery trunk.

Colic nodes:
a. Epicolic (on the colonic wall).
b. Paracolic (along the bowel wall).
c. Intermediate – a long colic arteries.
d. Preterminal – adjacent to SMA and IMA.

Perirectal nodes are seen close to the wall of rectum not in the wall.

53. a. False   b. True   c. False   d. True   e. True

Uterus measures 6–7 x 5 x 7 cm, 3 cm thickness.

The tube can extend for up to 10 cm from cornue infundibulum cervix measures 3–4 cm, canal measures 7–8 cm.

54. a. False   b. False   c. False   d. True   e. False

Fluid in the pouch of Douglas is very common in ectopic pregnancy and can be haemorrhage.

GIFT is gamete intrafallopian transfer and has increased the incidence of ectopic pregnancy.

55. a. False   b. True   c. True   d. True   e. True

Also with duplex system. Renal artery stenosis, renal tubular acidosis, horseshoe kidney, and Caroli's disease.

56. a. True   b. True   c. False   d. False   e. False

Reflux is the most common indication in children.

Micturition should take place in the left anterior oblique or right anterior oblique to visualise the lower ureter.

Dysuria can be due to trauma of catheter or secondary to infections.

Majority responds to simple analgesics. The bladder has more height than width in males. It can be funnel-shaped when patient is in erect position.

57. a. True   b. True   c. True   d. True   e. False

On CT scan, acute intrarenal infarction is seen as a wedge-shaped area of diminished renal enhancement (Lobar nephronia).

58. a. True   b. True   c. False   d. True   e. True

Acute renal failure characterised by sudden loss of the ability of the kidneys to excrete wastes, concentrate urine, conserve electrolytes, and maintain fluid balance.

59. a. True   b. False   c. True   d. True   e. False

Tumours that produce erythrocytemia are renal cell carcinoma, Wilm's, polycystic kidney disease, hepatoma, regenerating nodular hyperplasia, pheochromocytoma, Cushing's, adenoma, and cerebellar haemangiomapericytoma.

60. a. True   b. True   c. False   d. True   e. True

Nephrectomy can be radical or partial. The presence of adrenal or perinephric involvement outside Gerotas fasia is a contraindication for partial surgeries. Adrenal involvement occurs in 6% of tumours.

There is no evidence of that lymph glands resection improve prognosis. The incidence of metastasis is 50% higher in those with regional lymph node involvement. Renal venous involvement is seen in 20%.

61. a. True   b. False   c. True   d. True   e. True

Adrenal Adenoma
- Incidence in the population is 2–8%.

- Diagnosis is often made as an incidental finding on CT examinations.
- In patient with no known primary, an adrenal mass is almost always a benign adenoma.
- In a patient with a known neoplasm, especially lung cancer, an adrenal mass is problematic and diagnosing a metastasis versus and adenoma is critical for prognosis.

Imaging Findings
- CT
  - Size greater than 4 cm tend to be metastases or adrenal carcinoma—heterogenous appearance and irregular shape are malignant characteristics.
  - Homogenous and smooth are benign characteristics—intracellular lipid in adenoma results in low attenuation on CT.
  - Little intracytoplasmic fat in metastases results in high attenuation on non-enhanced CT.
  - Non-enhanced CT (NECT) – threshold 10 HU; sensitivity 79%, specificity 96%.
  - Contrast enhanced CT (CECT) – because majority of CT examinations in oncology use IV contrast, the % washout is useful after 10 minutes; adenoma have greater than 50% washout after 10 minutes; washout can be used on adrenal masses that measure > 10 HU on NECT; alternative is to do MR or PET.
- MR
  - Chemical shift – most sensitive method for differentiating adenomas from metastases; sensitivity 81–100%, specificity 94–100%; the difference in resonance rate of protons in fat and water is exploited in chemical shift.
    - Intracellular lipid and water in same voxel result in summation of signal on 'in-phase' and cancelling out of signal on 'out of phase'.
  - Spleen or muscle is used as an internal standard to visually quantify signal drop-off—liver is not a reliable standard because of steatosis.

62. a. False   b. False   c. False   d. True   e. True

Carcinoid Tumours Adenoma

- Low grade malignancies.
- About 10% metastasize.
- Most patients under 50 years.
- Most common primary lung tumour under age 16 years.
- Male to female ratio of 1:1.
- White to black 25:1.
- Neurosecretory production of serotonin ACTH and bradykinin.
- Salivary gland types: cylindromas, mucoepidermoid mixed.

Clinical Findings
- Haemoptysis 40–50%.
- Atypical asthma.
- Persistent cough.
- Recurrent pneumonia.
- Asymptomatic (10%).

Radiological chest x-ray finding include atelectasis or pneumonia or rarely emphysema.

Very few carcinoids of lung give rise to carcinoid syndrome, those that do always have widespread metastases to the liver.

Overall prognosis: 75% and 15 years survival.

Associated with Cushing's disease is rare.

63.	a. True	b. False	c. False	d. True	e. True
64.	a. True	b. True	c. False	d. True	e. True
65.	a. True	b. True	c. False	d. True	e. True
66.	a. True	b. True	c. True	d. False	e. True
67.	a. True	b. True	c. True	d. False	e. True
68.	a. False	b. True	c. True	d. True	e. True
69.	a. True	b. True	c. True	d. False	e. False

70. a. False   b. False   c. False   d. True   e. False

- Spasm is avoided by using warmed contrast.
- Balloon catheter should be inflated in the navicular fossa.
- The best procedure for demonstrating prostatic urethra is cystography.
- Urethrography is good for distal urethra.
- Supine 30 degrees LAO and RAO are done.
- Urethral fistula is best seen in voiding films.

71. a. True   b. True   c. True   d. True   e. False

- Filariasis is the commonest cause. Other causes include those which causes compression or narrowing of thoracic duct or fistula between renal tract and lymphatics, tuberculosis, trauma, surgery, lymphoma, and other neoplasms.

72. a. True   b. True   c. False   d. True   e. True

Bladder Rupture – Intraperitoneal
- Can be secondary to traumatic or iatrogenic injury.
- Five types of rupture:
  o Type I: Bladder contusion – most common form results from incomplete tear of bladder mucosa.
  o Type II: Intraperitoneal rupture – results from trauma to lower abdomen when bladder is distended; contrast is then seen in the paracolic gutters and between loops of small bowel.
  o Type III: Interstitial injury – rare, caused by a tear of the serosal surface, mural defect without extravasation will be seen.
  o Type IV: Extraperitoneal (most common) – almost always associated with pelvic surface, usually close to base of bladder anterolaterally, subdivided into:
    - Simple, with extraluminal contrast limited to perivesical space.
    - Complex, with extaluminal contrast extending to thigh, scrotum, and perineum.
  o Type V: Combined extra- and intraperitoneal rupture.
- Usually iatrogenic or secondary to penetrating injury.
- Blunt trauma more likely to result in intraperitoneal rupture in children than in adults.

- While extraperitoneal bladder rupture can be treated conservatively, intraperitoneal bladder rupture requires surgical repair.

Imaging Findings
- Diagnostic evaluation of bladder rupture includes voiding cystourethrography (VCUG) or CT scan
    o VCUG
- Bladder needs to fully distend and evaluation of post-voiding film essential.
- Plain film.
- 'Pear-shaped' bladder.
- Upward displacement of ileal loops—flame-shaped contrast extravasation into perivesical fat.
- US.
- 'Bladder within a bladder' = bladder surrounded by fluid collection.

73. a. True   b. True   c. True   d. True   e. False

74. a. True   b. True   c. False   d. True   e. False

MRI is not superior to CT in assessment of lymph nodal involvement. It is better than CT in differentiating nodes from collateral vessels which are seen as sign voids. They are not useful in differentiating bowel and nodal masses. MRI is not useful in detection small renal cancers, especially less than 1 cm and calcification. It is very useful in differentiating adrenal adenomas from metastasis. The accuracy in 98% for detection of adjacent visceral involvement.

Contrast enhanced spiral CT scan is still the best method of staging renal cell carcinoma and MRI is an adjunctive tool, especially for venous invasion.

75. a. True   b. False   c. True   d. True   e. False

76. a. False   b. True   c. True   d. True   e. True

Star-gazing fetus is fetal cervical hyperextension in breech presentation. Amelia is absence of a limb. Hemimelia is absence of the distal segment of a limb. Phocomelia is absence of the proximal segment of a limb. Symmelia is fusion of the limb in whole or in part (Mermaid).

77. a. True   b. True   c. False   d. False   e. True

Scar endometriosis is a term given to endometriosis occurring in a ceasarean section scar. It can occur at the skin, subcutaneous rectus muscle, interperitoneally, or uterine myometrium.
Some patient asymptomatic other constant pain. Usually single mass, rarely cystic.

78. a. True   b. True   c. True   d. False   e. True

79. a. True   b. True   c. True   d. False   e. False

80. a. False   b. False   c. True   d. False   e. False

Skene glands are paired paraurethral glands that connect with the anterior vagina at the introitus via a duct called skene ducts providing lubrication mainly at the time of orgasm. If the duct is obstruct, secretion build up lending to a fluid-filled mass and need surgical excision one MRI the mass seen in the anterior introitus containing proteinaceous fluid.

81. a. True   b. False   c. True   d. True   e. False

Amniotic fluid index (AFI) it is part of the fatal biophysical profile to estimate the amniotic fluid volume. Normal AFI values range from 5 to 25 cm. AFI between 8 and 18 cm is considered median AFI level is approximately 14 cm from week 20 to 35 cm after which the amniotic fluid begins to reduce. AFI less than 5–6cm is considered as oligohydraminos. AFI more than 20–24 cm is considered polyhydraminos.

82. a. True   b. True   c. False   d. False   e. True

83. a. False   b. True   c. True   d. True   e. False

84. a. True   b. False   c. False   d. False   e. True

85. a. True   b. True   c. True   d. False   e. False

86. a. True   b. True   c. False   d. True   e. True

87. a. False   b. False   c. True   d. False   e. True

Ureteritis cystica – rare and benign condition of the ureter and sometimes renal pelvis (pyelitis cystica) resulting from multiple fluid-containing submucosal cysts. Associated with chronic inflammation and diabetics with chronic and recurring urinary tract infections and may be associated with nephrolithiasis and chronic obstruction. The cysts result from degeneration of epithelial cells. Bilateral is possible. Most often found at 50–60 years of age. Usually asymptomatic.

Best diagnosed by cystoscopy, can be diagnosed by retrograde pyelogram or antegrade CT urography or intravenous pyelogram. It is not premalignant.

88. a. False   b. True   c. True   d. True   e. True

Hypoplastic limb, osteoporosis, pathological fracture, hydronephrosis, hydroureters, bladder outlet obstruction, spinal dysraphism, lacunar skull, hydrocephalus, and renal osteodystrophy.

89. a. True   b. False   c. True   d. False   e. False

90. a. True   b. False   c. True   d. True   e. True

Most common fusion abnormality of the kidney. Fusion is at the lower pole in 90% of cases. Complications includes uretropelvic junction obstruction, recurrent infections, calculus formation and increased incidence of Wilm's tumour, transitional cell carcinoma.

91. a. True   b. True   c. True   d. False   e. True

The osteoporosis in oat cell carcinoma is non-endocrinal steroid-producing tumour. Other endocrinal cause such as thyroid abnormality or pancreatic insufficiency. Adrenocortical abnormality, e.g., Cushing's syndrome. Hypogonadism cause, e.g., menopause, Turner's syndrome.

92. a. True   b. True   c. True   d. False   e. True

93. a. True   b. True   c. True   d. True   e. False

94. a. True   b. True   c. True   d. False   e. False

95. a. False   b. True   c. True   d. True   e. False

96. a. False   b. True   c. True   d. True   e. True

Widening of the presacral space is one of the diagnostic indicators of the disease involving pelvic pathology and rectal involvement.

The space measured on lateral radiographs at the level 0f S3/S4 disc level to the posterior wall of the rectum (on contrast study). The presacral space above 1.5 cm indicate abnormality either within the rectum e.g. inflammatory process or within the sacrum e.g. chordoma or in between within the soft tissue e.g. abscess.

97. a. True   b. True   c. True   d. False   e. True

Robert pelvis when there is hypoplasia of the sacral alae.

The Nagele pelvis is asymmetrical deformity of the inlet.

98. a. False   b. True   c. True   d. True   e. True

Epidermoid cyst of the Testicle
- Rare testicular lesion accounting for 1-2% of testicular tumors.
- Benign testicular tumor with no malignant potential.
- Most commonly, this lesion occurs in the 2nd-4th decades of life.
- Clinical presentation usually involves testicular enlargement or a palpable mass without other clinical symptoms.
- More common in the right testicle. There have been very rare cases of bilateral epidermoid cysts.

Ultrasound imaging findings
- Ultrasound is the study of choice.
- Ultrasound will show a round and well demarcated intratesticular mass.
- Internal heterogeneity, often with alternating hyperechoic and hyperechoic internal rings with an "onion skin" appearance.
- A hyperechoic center is often present.
- May have a hyperechoic or hypoechoic rim.
- Avascular on color imaging.

MRI Imaging findings
- Well demarcated intratesticular mass.
- T2 weighted imaging shows high signal intensity that may have low intensity internal foci and a low intensity rim.
- Absence of enhancement with contrast.

1. Features of epiploic appendagitis:
   a) Ascites.
   b) Dilated bowel loop locally.
   c) Constipation.
   d) Burning micturition.
   e) Abdominal pain and guarding.

2. In Killian-Jamieson diverticulum:
   a) It is a pulsion diverticulum.
   b) Arises from cervical oesophagus just above the cricopharyngeal muscle.
   c) Also called Zenker's diverticulum.
   d) May presented with recurrent aspiration pneumonia.
   e) Is premalignant.

3. In choledocal cyst:
   a) Well seen on a cutaneous transhepatic cholangioma.
   b) Type V is cystic dilation of the intrhepatic ducts.
   c) May be demonstrated on a Rose Bengal scan.
   d) Type I is rare.
   e) May displace the stomach to the left.

4. Macrocytic anaemia is associated with the following:
   a) Carcinoma of the stomach.
   b) Renal cell carcinoma.
   c) Bronchogenic carcinoma.
   d) Diverticular disease.
   e) Leukaemia.

5. Intramural hemorrhage occurs in:
   a) Leukemia.
   b) Crohn's disease.
   c) Ankylostoma duodenal.
   d) Trauma.
   e) Uremia.

6. Polydepsia occurs:
   a) Diabetes insipidus.
   b) Craniopharyngioma.
   c) Hypoparathyroidism.
   d) Pheocromocytoma.
   e) Diabetes mellitus.

7. The following are true in Crohn's disease:
   a) Associated with gallstone.
   b) Commonly involve the terminal ileum.
   c) Rarely involve the rectum.
   d) Continuous and superficial ulceration of the gut is a feature.
   e) Sclerossing cholangitis is common.

8. The following are true:
   a) If gastric ulcer is larger than 1 inch in diameter it is malignant.
   b) A mass in the stomach with an ulcer on, it is likely to be benign.
   c) Carcinoma of the gastric antrum causes spasms of the that region.
   d) Malignant gastric ulcer will not respond the medical treatment.
   e) Barium meal examination is the best way of telling of a DU has healed.

9. Prevertebral soft tissue mass in a child seen in:
   a) Goiter.
   b) Pharyngeal pouch.
   c) Chordoma.
   d) Cystic hyogroma.
   e) Neuroblastoma.

10. The following are true of congenital malrotation of the bowel:
    a) Is associated with asplenia.
    b) May present as intestinal obstruction.

c) The duodenal-jejunal flexure remains fixed in its normal position.
d) Small bowel is associated with large bowel volvulus.
e) Is associated with exomphalos.

11. In congenital diaphragmatic hernia:
a) More common on the right side.
b) Scaphoid abdomen.
c) Presentation at birth with severe respiratory distress.
d) Degree of lung hypoplasia.
e) Associated with cyanotic congenital heart disease.

12. Protein losing enteropathy is found:
a) Villous adenoma.
b) Uremia.
c) Intestinal lymphangiectasis.
d) Hodgkin's disease.
e) Mastocytosis.

13. Acute appendicitis, the following are true:
a) Common in Crohn's disease.
b) Common in carcinoid.
c) By ultrasound, the lumen is distended more than 6 mm in diameter with circumferential wall thickening.
d) Fecolith is rarely present.
e) It may be due to parasite.

14. Meconium ileus demonstrated:
a) Dilated colon on enema.
b) Peritoneal calcification.
c) Pancreatic calcification.
d) Pneumoperitonium.
e) Fluid levels on an erect abdominal film.

15. Glucagons administration, the following are true:
a) The stomach to dilate and duodenum to contact.
b) Improve overall bowels visualisation for patient underwent MR enterography examinations.
c) Hypotonic colon.
d) Nausea and vomiting are common.
e) Dysphagia.

16. Ascites is seen in the following in the neonates:
    a) Prune belly.
    b) Neuroblastoma.
    c) Congenital biliary atresia.
    d) Erythroblastosis fetalis.
    e) Obstructive uropathy.

17. The following are true regarding gastric polyp:
    a) Hyperplastic polyp is the most common type and associated with pernicious anaemia.
    b) Adenomatous polyp is associated with juvenile polyposis.
    c) Retention polyp is associated with Cronkhite-Canada syndrome.
    d) Gardener's syndrome associated with villous polyp.
    e) Bleeding is common.

18. In porcelain gallbladder:
    a) Commonly in hyperthyroidism.
    b) CT is more sensitive than conventional radiographs.
    c) Easy missed by ultrasound examination.
    d) About 25% develops carcinoma of gallbladder.
    e) It may mistaken by a large gallstone with peripheral calcification in contracted gallbladder.

19. In diabetes the following are true:
    a) Calcification of the fallopian tubes is characteristics.
    b) Increased incidence of congenital malformation in diabetic mothers.
    c) Increased incidence in pancreatic carcinoma.
    d) In diabetic ketoacidosis gastric dilatation may occur.
    e) Cardiomyopathy is a feature.

20. The following are true in obstructive jaundice:
    a) Usually associated with airobilia.
    b) May be associated with Klatskin's tumour.
    c) Mirizzi syndrome is a recognise cause.
    d) Ascaris may be the cause.
    e) The common bile duct is dilated measures more than 7 mm in most of the cases of obstructive jaundice.

21. In superior mesenteric artery syndrome:
    a) Compressed 2nd part of the duodenum.
    b) The angle between the aorta and superior mesenteric artery is decreased to 45° in the disease.
    c) The compression is relieved by turning the patient to the left duodenum.
    d) A transverse linear compression defect can be seen over the duodenum on barium study.
    e) The duodenum is dilated proximal to the site of compression significantly.

22. Dysphagia is a symptom of:
    a) Arnold-chiari malformation.
    b) Linitis plastic.
    c) Pancreatic carcinoma.
    d) Bronchogenic carcinoma
    e) Giant left atrium.

23. The following are associated with:
    a) Thymoma and erythraemia.
    b) Asplenia and congenital heart disease.
    c) Neuro-enteric cyst and coronal cleft vertebra.
    d) Multiple osteoma and chronic diarrhoea.
    e) Diverticulosis and Sacroilitis.

24. In typhilitis:
    a) Is neutropenic colitis of the right colon.
    b) Associated with leukaemia.
    c) Typically affects the paediatric population.
    d) CT scan is the diagnostic modality of choice.
    e) Surgically treated.

25. The following are true in related to splenomegaly:
    a) Enlarged in repeated haemodialysis.
    b) Splenomegaly may cause left hydronephrosis.
    c) Auto-splenectomy can be seen in sickle cell disease.
    d) High risk of leukaemia after splenectomy.
    e) Splenic index more than 140 cm^3 indicate splenomegaly.

26. In tuberculosis of the ileum:
    a) Mycobacterium tuberculosis and yersina enterocolitica are the most commonly involve the terminal ileum.
    b) Commonly accompanied by adenopathy locally.
    c) Commonly accompanied by pulmonary tuberculosis.
    d) Can give the same radiological appearances and complications of that in Crohn's disease.
    e) Treated by steroids and anti-tubercles drugs usually.

27. In ectopic gallbladder:
    a) Premalignant.
    b) Displaced to the left side.
    c) Usually isolated finding.
    d) Associated with Riedel lobe of the liver.
    e) Associated with multiple gallstones usually.

28. In ischemic cholitis:
    a) Commonly affected the left side of the colon.
    b) Sparing the rectum.
    c) Oral contraceptive is predisposing factor.
    d) Thumb printing ulcer can be seen by barium enema.
    e) Premalignant in chronic cases.

29. Causes of liver cirrhosis:
    a) α 1 antitrypsin deficiency.
    b) Wilson disease.
    c) Schistosomes.
    d) Contraceptive pill.
    e) Methotrexate overdose.

30. Intramural haemorrhage occurs in:
    a) Leukaemia.
    b) Crohn's disease.
    c) Ankylostoma duodenal.
    d) Trauma.
    e) Warfarin toxicity.

31. In Systemic Mastocytosis is associated with:
    a) Skin involvement.
    b) Gastrointestinal tract is rarely affected.
    c) Osteosclerotic bony changes.

d) Alcohol consumption may precipitate the symptoms.
e) Peptic ulcer is common.

32. Peptic esophagitis in infants:
    a) Is frequently cured by medical treatment alone.
    b) Deep penetrating ulceration may develop.
    c) May present as failure to thrive.
    d) Commonest cause of hematemesis in children.
    e) Associated with sideropenic webs.

33. In cholangiocarcinoma:
    a) Distant metastases are common.
    b) Arise from the lining of the bile ducts.
    c) May called Klatskin tumour.
    d) Is often fatal condition.
    e) Associated with Mirizzi syndrome.

34. In adult pyloric stenosis:
    a) Associated with achalasia.
    b) Commonly due to duodenal ulcer.
    c) May be due to ectopic pancreatic nodule.
    d) May be due to Hodgkin's disease.
    e) Gastric outlet obstruction is rare.

35. Bowel wall on CT scan:
    a) Normally not enhanced after the administration of IV contrast medium.
    b) Normal small bowel wall thickness is up to 3 mm despite luminal distention.
    c) Normal large bowel wall thickness is up to 5 mm when the wall is contracted.
    d) Most of the bowel malignant tumours presented as multiple, segmental, and diffuse thickening of the bowel wall.
    e) Small bowel lymphoma is typically shows as a segmental distribution.

36. Annular pancreas is associated with:
    a) Congenital heart disease.
    b) Mongolism.
    c) Esophageal atresia.

d) Turner's syndrome.
e) Malrotation of gut.

37. Multiple air / fluid levels may be shown on the erect abdomen in:
a) Irritable colon syndrome.
b) Celiac disease.
c) Small bowel diverticulosis.
d) Pneumatosis intestinalis.
e) Gastric enteritis in infants.

38. An enema using water-soluble contrast media is useful therapeutic procedure in:
a) Gastroenteritis.
b) Meconium ileus.
c) Hirschsprung's disease.
d) Intussusception.
e) Ulcerative colitis.

39. The following features may be present in meconium ileus:
a) Fluid levels on plain erect abdomen.
b) Calcification in the peritoneum.
c) The colon appears dilated on barium enema.
d) Pneumoperitoneum.
e) Normal abdominal radiograph.

40. Features of necrotizing entero-colitis in infants include:
a) Gas in the portal vessels.
b) Pneumoperitoneum.
c) Pneumatosis coli.
d) Distended gas-filled bowel.
e) Gas in the biliary tree.

41. The following statements are true:
a) In the neonate, neuroblastoma is more common than Wilm's tumour.
b) Lung secondaries are more common in neuroblastatoma than in Wilm's tumour.
c) In neonate, neuroblastoma metastasizes to the liver most commonly.
d) Neuroblastoma is a recognised cause of infantile proptosis.
e) Calcification is seen in over 70% of primary neuroblastoma.

42. In esophageal webs:
    a) Common middle-aged men.
    b) Associated with iron deficiency anaemia.
    c) May be multiple.
    d) Are best seen by barium swallow.
    e) Are frequently asymptomatic.

43. In Zinker diverticulum:
    a) Compressible neck mass.
    b) Upper oesophageal dysphagia.
    c) Halitosis.
    d) Associated with hiatal hernia.
    e) Commonly in young men.

44. Bile-stained vomiting and abdominal distension in neonates may be seen:
    a) Septicemia.
    b) Congenital pyloric stenosis.
    c) Axial rotation of the stomach.
    d) Hirschsprung's disease.
    e) A meconium plug.

45. Solitary splenic calcification seen in:
    a) Epidermoid cyst.
    b) Sickle cell anaemia.
    c) Dermoid.
    d) Mucoviscidosis (fibrocystic disease of pancreas).
    e) Polysplenia.

46. Liver calcification seen:
    a) Intrahepatic gallbladder.
    b) Gamma.
    c) Portal vein thrombosis.
    d) Histocytosis.
    e) Hemochromatosis.

47. The following are features of meconium ileus:
    a) A dilated colon.
    b) Oral water soluble contrast is contraindicated.
    c) Displace the meconium usually occurs in 48 hours.

d) A speckled appearance of the intestinal contents on plain radiograph.
e) Fluid levels are not a prominent feature.

48. In tuberose sclerosis:
    a) May cause spontaneous pneumothorax.
    b) Frequently causes cerebellar calcification.
    c) May produce small cortical cysts in the kidneys.
    d) Is a cause of café-au-lait spots.
    e) Affected patients are of normal mentality.

49. Gastric dilatation occurs in:
    a) Aerophagia.
    b) Morphine administration.
    c) Constipation.
    d) Lead poisoning.
    e) Uremia.

50. In Interstitial emphysema of the stomach:
    a) Phlegmonous gastritis.
    b) Pancreatitis.
    c) Hirschsprung's disease.
    d) Necrotizing gastro enterocolitis.
    e) Pneumatosis cystoides.

51. In neonate, the double bubble sign on erect film of abdomen seen:
    a) Annular pancreas.
    b) Duodenal atresia.
    c) Ladd bands.
    d) Midgut volvulus.
    e) Hirschsprung's disease.

52. Intestinal polyps in a child is a feature of the following:
    a) Neurofibromatosis.
    b) Turcot syndrome.
    c) Cronknite-Canada syndrome.
    d) Whipple's disease.
    e) Osler Weber disease.

53. Extrinsic defect of the cervical oesophagus may be due:
    a) Parathyroid tumour.
    b) Plummer-Vinson syndrome.
    c) Spinal spur.
    d) Leiomyoma.
    e) Vegas nerve tumour.

54. In a neonate with intestinal obstruction and bilous vomiting, the following should be suspected:
    a) Pyloric stenosis.
    b) Malrotation.
    c) Ectopic pancreas.
    d) Intestinal polyposis.
    e) Intussusception.

55. Gas in the biliary tree occurs in:
    a) Ascariasis.
    b) Early carcinoma of pancreas.
    c) Within the gallstone.
    d) Late pyloric stenosis.
    e) Cholangitis.

56. In Hirschsprung's disease:
    a) Commonly in female.
    b) Bilious vomiting is a feature.
    c) Impaired mental functioning.
    d) Usually recto sigmoid involved.
    e) May involve all the colon.

57. In Boerhaave syndrome the following are true:
    a) Spontaneous rupture of the cervical diverticulum.
    b) Intramural diverticulum is main cause.
    c) Due to sudden rise of intra luminal esophageal pressure.
    d) Typically the rupture occurs in the left side of the lower oesophagus.
    e) A right-sided pleural effusion is often visible on chest radiographs.

58. In para esophageal hernia:
    a) Cardia is displaced above the diaphragm.
    b) Commonly reducible.

c) Associated with gastric ulcer.
d) Premalignant.
e) Associated with reflux.

59. In wandering spleen:
    a) Associated with lax abdominal wall.
    b) Commonly in women.
    c) No flow within the spleen on Doppler ultrasound.
    d) Heavy calcification is almost always seen.
    e) Associated with GIT bleeding.

60. Disordered oesophageal moltility may occur as a feature of:
    a) Klippe-feil syndrome.
    b) Ehlers-Danlos syndrome.
    c) Gaucher's disease.
    d) Scleroderma.
    e) Riley Day Syndrome (Familial Dysautonia).

61. Adrenal calcification may occur in:
    a) Adreno congital syndrome.
    b) Niemann-Pick syndrome.
    c) Disseminated intravascular coagulation.
    d) Wolman's syndrome.
    e) Cushing's syndrome.

62. The following statements are true:
    a) In meconium ileus the colon is of normal calibre.
    b) In meconium plug syndrome the colon is of normal calibre.
    c) A microcolon is present in ileal atresia.
    d) Duodenal atresia is associated with a microcolon.
    e) There is an association between diabetic mothers and microcolon.

63. Dilatation of the duodenum in adults seen in:
    a) Strongyloidiasis.
    b) Hirschsprung's disease.
    c) Acute pancreatitis.
    d) Dermatomyositis.
    e) Whipple's disease.

64. There is a well-recognised association between:
    a) Mongolism and duodenal atresia.
    b) Duodenal atresia and ileal atresia.
    c) Hirschprung's and hip dysplasia.
    d) Oesophageal atresia and duodenal atresia.
    e) Duodenal atresia and malrotation.

65. Pseudomyxoma peritonei may follow lesion arising in:
    a) Appendix.
    b) Ovary.
    c) Gallbladder.
    d) Pancreas.
    e) Uterus.

66. A posterior impression on the oesophagus is seen in:
    a) Aberrant right subclavian artery.
    b) Aberrant left main pulmonary artery.
    c) Patent ductus arteriosus.
    d) Coartation.
    e) SVC obstruction.

67. On 10th post abdominal operative day the following help to differentiate subphrenic abscess from pulmonary infarct:
    a) Raised hemidiaphragm.
    b) Pleural effusion.
    c) Gas under one hemidiaphragm.
    d) Extrinsic mass indenting gastric fundus.
    e) Paralysed hemidiaphragm on screening.

68. In intrahepatic cholangiocarcinoma is:
    a) The 2nd most common primary hepatic tumour after hepatoma.
    b) Commonly in young female.
    c) Marked homogeneous delay enhancement on CT scan.
    d) Large central homogeneous hypointense mass on T1W1.
    e) New vascularity in about 50% on angiography.

69. Radiological features of small bowel carcinoids:
    a) Mucosal elevation.
    b) Calcified mesenteric mass.
    c) Crowding of folds.

d) Hernia.
e) Intussusception.

70. In chilaiditi syndrome:
    a) Due to intestinal obstruction.
    b) Associated with emphysema.
    c) Indicating previous abdominal surgery.
    d) Almost always asymptomatic.
    e) Indicating worm infestation.

71. Clinical significant of protein loss may occur:
    a) Radation entiritis.
    b) Villous adenoma.
    c) Whipple's disease.
    d) Ulcerative colitis.
    e) Cascade stomach.

72. The following are true in esophageal stent:
    a) The aim only to maintain patency of the esophageal lumen.
    b) MRI recommended within the first week after stent placement.
    c) Migration and in folding of the device occur immediately after placement.
    d) Increase incidence of esophageal cancer.
    e) Mass at the ends of the stent commonly indicating mucosal edema.

73. Raised amylase is seen in:
    a) Cholecystitis.
    b) Perforated peptic ulcer.
    c) Ischemic colitis.
    d) Renal colic.
    e) Acute pancreatitis.

74. Drugs induced paralytic ileus (acute non obstructive small bowel distention):
    a) Morphine.
    b) Probanthine.
    c) Hexmethonium.
    d) Methygerside.
    e) L-dopa.

75. Henoch-Schonlein Purpura is associated with:
    a) Renal failure.
    b) Erosive arthropathy.
    c) Intersusseption.
    d) Subarachnoid haemorrhage.
    e) Intestinal haemorrhage.

76. Pernicious anaemia is associated with:
    a) Atrophy of gastric mucosa.
    b) Jejunal mucosal atrophy.
    c) Gastric ulceration.
    d) Gastric polyposis.
    e) Increase gastric peristalsis.

77. Intussusception the following are true:
    a) Red current jelly stools usually only after > 48 hours duration.
    b) Palpable abdominal mass is about 60%.
    c) Self-limiting disease.
    d) Located in the splenic flexure more than the hepatic flexure.
    e) Necrotizing enterocolitis is predisposing factor.

78. The following are true in necrotizing enterocolitis:
    a) Perforation is rare.
    b) Prognosis is good.
    c) Football sign is always present.
    d) Pneumatosis may be seen in the stomach wall.
    e) Gas in the biliary system on plain radiogram is a feature.

79. In Cushing's syndrome:
    a) Males are more affected than females.
    b) Hyperplasia of the adrenal gland is more common than adenoma.
    c) Carcinoma of the adrenal gland is more common than adenoma.
    d) Associated with basophil adenoma.
    e) Best diagnosed by unenhanced CT scan of abdomen.

80. Peptic esophagitis in infants:
    a) Is frequently cured by medical treatment alone.
    b) Deep penetrating ulceration may develop.
    c) Present as failure to thrive.

d) Commonest cause of hematemesis in children.
e) Associated with sideropenic webs.

81. The following are causes of megacolon:
    a) Obesity.
    b) Toxic colon due to ulcerative colitis.
    c) Crohn's disease.
    d) Chilaiditis syndrome.
    e) Turcot syndrome.

82. The following are associated with:
    a) Erythema nodosum and Hodgkin's disease.
    b) Basal cell nevi and jaw cysts.
    c) Polyostotic fibrous dysplasia and nevi.
    d) Hydatid cysts and hepatoma.
    e) Hyperparathyroidism and pancreatitis.

83. Coeliac disease is associated:
    a) Increased malignancy.
    b) Jaundice.
    c) Diverticulosis of the jejunum.
    d) Rapid transit time.
    e) Edematous primary mucosal folds.

84. In cecal volvulus the following are true:
    a) Associated with horseshoe kidney.
    b) Associated with diverticulitis in the left colon.
    c) Can be confidently diagnosed by plain abdomen.
    d) Commonly on old females.
    e) Beak configuration to end of barium column seen by barium enema examination.

85. The following point in favour to malignancy in polyp of bowel:
    a) Greater than 1 cm in size.
    b) Irregular in outline.
    c) Multiple polyps.
    d) Increase in size.
    e) Pedunculated.

86. In gastric diverticula:
    a) Always acquired.
    b) Usually asymptomatic.
    c) Usually missed by barium meal study.
    d) May be associated with an increased risk of malignancy.
    e) Pneumoperitonium indicating perforation.

87. Adrenal calcification the following are true:
    a) Caused by Addison's disease.
    b) Associated with Wolman's disease.
    c) Neuroblastoma is recognised cause in infancy.
    d) May indicate phechromocytoma.
    e) Calcification seen within 1st week of the haemorrhage.

88. The following are true in carcinoma of the colon:
    a) Peak age 50–70 years.
    b) Commonly diagnosed confidently by barium enema alone.
    c) Rarely spread to the liver.
    d) Scirrhous carcinoma infiltrating type is much more than annular constricting type (apple-core lesion).
    e) Pneumatosis intestinalis is recognised complication.

89. Ideal barium concentration used for different parts examination for GI tract:
    a) Barium meal 250% weight/volume.
    b) Barium swallow 100% weight/volume.
    c) Follow through 200% weight/volume.
    d) Small large bowel enema 60% weight/volume.
    e) Large bowel barium enema 250% weight/volume.

90. In esophageal atresia and tracheoesophageal fistula:
    a) Can be suggested the diagnosis on prenatal ultrasound.
    b) H-type diagnosed within the first 24 hours of life usually.
    c) Imperforated anus is common association.
    d) CT scan is the examination of choice.
    e) 13 pairs of ribs are commonly present.

91. In carcinoid tumour of the small bowel:
    a) Associated with scleroderma.
    b) Associated with intestinal obstruction.
    c) Most common primary tumour of the small bowel.

d) Most of appendicular carcinoid is malignant.
e) Solitary liver metastasis is common.

92. In emphysematous cholecystitis:
    a) Jaundice is common.
    b) Can be diagnosed confidently by conventional radiography.
    c) Air in gallbladder wall is diagnostic feature.
    d) Cholelithiasis is rare.
    e) Acute infection of gallbladder caused by gas-forming organism.

93. Hodgkin's disease the following are true:
    a) Alcohol-induced pain.
    b) Sparring the spleen.
    c) Painful lymphadenopathy is usual.
    d) Localised pruritus is common.
    e) Represent 5% of all lymphoma.

94. In liver haemangioma the following are true:
    a) It is premalignant.
    b) Associated with thrombocytopenia.
    c) Associated with haemangioma in other organs.
    d) The most common benign liver tumour.
    e) May enlarge during pregnancy.

95. Infantile hypertrophic pyloric stenosis the following are true:
    a) Non-bilious projectile vomiting is a feature.
    b) Positive family history.
    c) Self-limiting disease.
    d) Mean age 3 years.
    e) Palpable olive-shaped mass.

96. The following are true in ileal atresia:
    a) Post-op functional obstruction.
    b) Ileal atresia much more common than stenosis.
    c) It may be multiple.
    d) Barium enema is indicated.
    e) Barium meal and follow through is advised.

97. The following are true in hepatoblastoma:
    a) May be present at birth.
    b) More common in girls.

c) Serum alpha-fetaprotein levels are elevated in more than 90% of patients.
d) Chemotherapy may be of advantage.
e) Associated with hemihyperatrophy.

98. The following are true in cirrhosis:
a) Common in cystic fibrosis.
b) In children alpha-1 antitrypsin deficiency may be the cause.
c) Hepatocellular carcinoma is rare.
d) Oesophageal variceal bleeding is rare in advance cirrhosis.
e) Associated with Paget's disease.

99. The following are true in pneumoperitonium:
a) 1–2 ml free intraperitoneal air can be visible on an upright chest film.
b) CT scan is best modality for demonstrating free intraperitoneal air.
c) Riglers sign (double wall sign) is meant air around the wall of the gallbladder.
d) Thin patient take long time to absorb air after surgery.
e) In newborn may indicate complicated meconium peritonitis.

100. In Whipple's disease:
a) More common in female.
b) Caused by gram negative bacteria.
c) Arthritis procedes intestinal disease in 50%.
d) Generalised lympadenopathy is seen in 50%.
e) Foamy macrophages in submucosa with PAS positive material is characteristic appearance.

101. Thickened, irregular folds valvulae conniventes are seen in:
a) Carcinoid.
b) Zollinger-Ellison syndrome.
c) Giardiasis.
d) Radiotherapy.
e) Celiac disease.

102. Chronic intestinal pseudo-obstruction is caused by:
a) SLE.
b) Hypothyroidism.
c) Diverticulosis.

d) Blind loop syndrome.
e) Mickles diverticulum.

103. The following are true in intestinal obstruction in children:
    a) Commonly due to Hirschsprung's disease.
    b) Hypertrophic pyloric stenosis is commonly in the first 3 months.
    c) Ileocolic intussusception is commonly at about 1 year of age.
    d) Appendicitis is recognised cause of intestinal obstruction in children.
    e) Bilious vomiting indicates high intestinal obstruction.

104. In focal nodular hyperplasia:
    a) Is the 2nd most common benign hepatic tumour.
    b) It is a benign congenital hamartomatous malformation.
    c) Commonly asymptomatic female in 3rd–4th decades of life.
    d) Haemorrhage and necrosis are common.
    e) Stellate fibrous scars are common.

105. In Mallory-Weiss tear:
    a) Common near the gastroesophageal junction.
    b) Seen in cirrhotic liver.
    c) History of vomiting is always present.
    d) The tear is multiple in majority.
    e) Transverse orientation.

106. In portal venous gas:
    a) Feature of necrotizing enterocolitis in children.
    b) Feature of Erythroblastosis fetalis.
    c) Iatrogenic.
    d) Associated with chronic obstructive lung disease.
    e) Air in the portal veins are more central in location.

107. In candida esophagitis:
    a) Odynophagia.
    b) Associated with scleroderma.
    c) Endoscopy is contraindicated.
    d) More fulminant form is more often associated with diabetes mellitus.
    e) Trachea-esophageal fistula is common complication in severe cases.

108. In achalasia cardia:
    a) Diagnosis is not made in the absence of a dilated oesophagus.
    b) Mimic malignancy.
    c) Carcinoma is a complication.
    d) Candida esophagitis is associated.
    e) Recurrent chest infections are common.

109. Gastrografin is better than barium because:
    a) It is cheaper.
    b) It is denser than barium.
    c) It shows the mucosal pattern better.
    d) It is less toxic if inhaled into the lungs.
    e) It is better absorbed from aerous surfaces.

110. The following are true of Cushing's disease:
    a) Associated with bronchial carcinoma.
    b) More common in men than in women.
    c) Associated with hypercalcemia.
    d) Associated with Islet cell tumour of pancreas.
    e) Associated with widding of mediastriium on PA chest x-ray.

111. The side effects of Buscopan (Hyoscine-N-Butylbromide 10 mg) include the following:
    a) Blurred vision.
    b) Bradycardia.
    c) Difficulty in micturition.
    d) Allergic response.
    e) Massive gastric dilatation.

112. Hernias of the abdomen the following are true:
    a) Ritcher's hernia contains the Meckel's diverticulum.
    b) Spigelian hernia happens through the rectus abdominis.
    c) Litter's hernia is blind ending tubular structure arising from antimesentric border of small bowel and extending into inguinal sac.
    d) Inguinal hernia is the most common hernia in female.
    e) Anterior peritoneal hernia is through a defect in the levator ani.

113. Giant haemangioma of the liver the following are true:
    a) Must be longer than 5 cm.
    b) Mostly asymptomatic.

c) Associated with Kasbach-Merritt syndrome.
d) Dynamic contrast-enhanced MRI of the abdomen is diagnostic.
e) Angiography demonstrates snowy tree appearance.

114. Feature of Whipple's disease:
    a) Dilatation of small bowel.
    b) Rigid folds.
    c) Rapid transit time.
    d) Thick folds.
    e) Small nodules.

115. In esophageal web:
    a) Associated with Plummer-Vinson syndrome.
    b) Associated with epidermolysis bullosa dystrophica.
    c) Usually fin in the infants.
    d) Located in the mid-third of the oesophagus.
    e) Premalignant.

116. In splenosis:
    a) Presence of splenic tissue in abnormal locations after splenic injury.
    b) In thoracic splenosis the patient may present with pleurisy or recurrent haemoptysis.
    c) Diagnosis confirmed by Tc-99m heat-damaged erythrocytes based on specific uptake of the radioactive isotope by splenic tissue.
    d) The presence of pleural nodules with a history of injury to the diaphragm and spleen should arouse suspicion of splenosis.
    e) Congenital variety associated with dextrocardia.

117. In liver metastases:
    a) Most liver metastases are single.
    b) Liver function testes tend to be specific.
    c) The most common primary sites for metastatic lesions in adults is gastrointestinal malignancies.
    d) Carcinoids metastasis is hypovascular.
    e) CT is the most sensitive technique for the detection of liver metastases.

118. Which are true:
    a) Bile salts are secreted by the gallbladder.
    b) Bile salts are absorbed in the terminal ileum.
    c) Pancreas divism is the most common congenital variant of the pancreatic anatomy.
    d) Acro-osteolysis in polyvinyl chloride osteolysis.
    e) Hypertelorism and mongolism.

119. In accessory pancreatic rests:
    a) Occur in fundus.
    b) Frequently undergo malignant change.
    c) May cause entero-enteric intussusception.
    d) May cause GI bleeding.
    e) May cause gastric outlet obstruction in neonate.

120. Anterior abdominal hernia includes:
    a) Ritcher hernia.
    b) Littre hernia.
    c) Foramen of Winslow.
    d) Epigastric hernia.
    e) Spigelian hernia.

121. Mucocele of the appendix may be associated with:
    a) Presented as appendicitis.
    b) Pseudomyxoma peritonei.
    c) Common in pregnancy.
    d) High attenuation on CT scan.
    e) Associated with carcinoid.

122. Barium enema in cathartic colon the following are true:
    a) Usually involves colon distal to splenic flexure.
    b) Patulous ileoceccal valve.
    c) Pseudopolyps formation of the colon.
    d) More haustration.
    e) Skip lesion.

123. In peritoneal mesothelioma:
    a) Associated with asbestos exposure.
    b) Associated with paraneoplastic syndrome.
    c) Omental caking seen on CT scan.

    d) MRI shows peritoneal masses demonstrate intermediate signal on T1; low high signal T2.
    e) Lung metastasis is early.

124. In diverticulosis of the colon:
    a) Almost always involves sigmoid.
    b) Never involve the rectum.
    c) May involve the entire colon.
    d) Commonly associated with Marfan's syndrome.
    e) More common in industrialized nation.

125. In gastroschisis:
    a) Herniation of abdominal content through a small defect in the abdominal wall.
    b) Usually involve the large bowel.
    c) Antenatal ultrasound is the study of choice.
    d) The abdominal defect located to the right of the umbilicus.
    e) Associated with Down syndrome.

126. Misty mesentery sign seen in:
    a) Mesenteric panniculitis.
    b) Sarcoidosis.
    c) Cirrhosis.
    d) Hypoalbuminemia.
    e) Haemorrhage.

127. In HIV esophagitis:
    a) Candidiasis is more common pathogens than herpes simplex virus.
    b) Multiple large ulcers more than 1 cm present on esophagram is usual.
    c) Endoscopy is contraindicated.
    d) Herpes usually produces multiple, small superficial ulcers without plaques, usually in the mid to upper oesophagus.
    e) Dysphasia and odynophagia are common symptoms with advanced HIV.

128. Radiation enteritis the following are true:
    a) Is due to endarteritis.
    b) Affects men more than women.
    c) More likely after abdominal surgery.

d) Affects 50% of these who have irradiation to the abdomen.
e) Commonly results in fistula formation.

129. Protein losing enteropathy is found:
    a) Villous adenoma.
    b) Uremia.
    c) Intestinal lymphangiectasis.
    d) Hodgkin's disease.
    e) Sarcoid.

130. The following are true in villous adenoma of the colon:
    a) Situated in the rectum.
    b) Severe hypoalbuminaemia.
    c) Don't coated easily by barium enema.
    d) Associated with ulcerative colitis.
    e) Associated with Crohn's disease.

131. Double bubble sign on erect plain abdomen x-ray typically seen in:
    a) Congenital pyloric stenosis.
    b) Duodenal atresia.
    c) Meckels diverticulum.
    d) Midgut volvulus.
    e) Annular pancreas.

132. CT scan of traumatic abdomen may be true:
    a) High-density intraperitoneal fluid (30–60 H) may be the only sign of injury.
    b) High attenuation fluid (80–130 H) is a sign of active bleeding.
    c) Free air in the peritoneal cavity is extremely rare.
    d) Subcapsular hematomas are usually crescent shaped.
    e) Free contrast agent in the peritoneal cavity is a sign of intraperitoneal bladder rupture or bowel perforation.

133. In interstitial emphysema of the stomach:
    a) Phlegmonous gastritis.
    b) Pneumatosis cystoides.
    c) Gastroscopy.
    d) Crohn's disease.
    e) Post-freezing gastritis.

134. In cholecystitis:
    a) Jackstone calculus.
    b) Mercedes-Benz sign.
    c) Popcorn calcification.
    d) Rice grain calcifications.
    e) Distended gallbladder, thickening of the wall and gallstones.

135. Risk factors in cholecystitis:
    a) Biliary sludge.
    b) Obesity.
    c) Pregnancy.
    d) Hyperparathyroidism.
    e) Crohn's disease.

136. In porcelain gallbladder:
    a) Premalignant.
    b) Asymptomatic usually.
    c) Associated with chronic cholecystitis.
    d) Associated with pancreatitis.
    e) Biliary obstruction is a feature.

137. Radiological feature of acute cholecystitis:
    a) Thickening of the gallbladder wall more than 3 mm.
    b) Distended gallbladder lumen greater than 5 cm.
    c) Air-fluid level in the gallbladder lumen.
    d) Pericholecystic fluid.
    e) Gastric dilatation.

138. CT scan finding in complicated acute cholecystitis:
    a) Air in the wall of the gallbladder.
    b) Decrease in bile density below 10 H.
    c) Free air in the abdomen.
    d) Stone in the terminal ilium.
    e) Halo of subserosal edema in the gallbladder.

139. In Lye stricture:
    a) Hoarseness may be present.
    b) Epigastric tenderness is common.
    c) Induce emesis is helpful in acute stage.
    d) Sore throat is almost always present.
    e) CT scan of neck, an immediate investigation.

140. Pneumatosis intestinal is associated with:
    a) Emphysematous cholecystitis.
    b) Emphysematous cystitis.
    c) Emphysematous gastritis.
    d) Necrotizing enterocolitis.
    e) Mainly sub mucosal.

141. Colon (cut off) sign seen:
    a) Pancreatitis.
    b) Hirschsprung's disease.
    c) Carcinoma of the colon.
    d) Mesenteric ischemia.
    e) Crohn's disease.

142. The following statements are true:
    a) Abuse of cathartics and pseudodiverticula of the colon.
    b) Sclerosing cholangitis and ulcerative colitis.
    c) Myasthenia gravia and myelomatosis.
    d) Steroid therapy and septal-B-lines on a chest radiography.
    e) The MRI imaging in multiple sclerosis will shows that the lesion in the white matter.

143. The following are true in oesphageal atresia:
    a) Frequently associated with tracheo-oesphageal fistula.
    b) Associated with annular pancreas.
    c) Associated with anal atresia.
    d) Fluoroscopy with water soluble contrast study is contra indicating in the 1st week of life.
    e) The fetus may appear growth restricted on antenatal ultrasound.

144. In toxic mega colon:
    a) Altered mental status
    b) Diagnosed test by barium enema double contrast.
    c) Transverse diameter of the transverse colon is more than 6 cm.
    d) Perforation is rare complication.
    e) Ascitis is common.

145. In duodenal Diverticulum:
    a) Peak incidence in 5th–6th decade.
    b) 90–95% is asymptomatic.
    c) Arise from medial wall (mesentric side) of duodenal sweep most commonly.

d) Premalignant.
e) Associated with iron deficiency anaemia.

146. GasLess abdomen in adult on plain radiograph seen in:
    a) Alcoholic patient
    b) Acute pancreatitis.
    c) Pyloric obstruction.
    d) Always abnormal.
    e) Closed-loop obstruction.

147. GasLess abdomen in a newborn may indicate:
    a) Tracheo-oesophageal fistula.
    b) Congenital diaphragmatic hernia.
    c) Always abnormal.
    d) Complete pyloric obstruction.
    e) Duodenal atresia.

148. Large abdominal gas pocket can be seen on plain abdomen in:
    a) Emphysematous cystitis.
    b) Blind loop syndrome.
    c) Physometria.
    d) Aerophagia.
    e) Syringomyelia.

149. Pancreatic calcification seen in:
    a) Kwashiorkor.
    b) Zollinger-Ellison syndrome.
    c) Acute pancreatitis.
    d) Alcoholic pancreatitis.
    e) Hypoparathyroidism.

150. Extrinsic defect of the cervical oesophagus seen in:
    a) Spinal spur.
    b) Pulmmer-Vinson syndrome.
    c) Aneurysm of the vertebral artery.
    d) Buckling of the carotid artery.
    e) Parathyroid adenoma.

151. Enlarged papilla of vater seen in:
    a) Sarcoidosis.
    b) Strongyloidosis.

c) Calculus.
d) Zollinger-Ellison syndrome.
e) Cholesterol polyp.

152. Blind loop syndrome that may give rise to malabsorption:
    a) Diverticulosis of small bowel.
    b) Duplication of bowel.
    c) Malroatation of bowel.
    d) Meckel's diverticulum.
    e) Post-operative gastroileostomy.

153. Thickened folds in the duodenum seen in:
    a) Cardiac failure.
    b) Achalasia of cardia.
    c) Pernicious anaemia.
    d) Zollinger-Ellison syndrome.
    e) Hypertrophy of Brunner's glands.

154. Thickening of the valvulae conniventes of the small bowel seen in:
    a) Mastocytosis.
    b) Pernicious anaemia.
    c) Anticoagulants.
    d) Whipple's disease.
    e) Giardiasis.

155. The following are true in desmoid tumour:
    a) More seen in women.
    b) Metastasis to the lungs commonly.
    c) When multiple, neurofibromatosis should be considered.
    d) The neck and chest are the common site.
    e) Response to chemotherapy.

156. Conditions associated with hemihypertrophy:
    a) Medullary sponge kidney.
    b) Wilm's tumour.
    c) Hypospadias.
    d) Medulloblastoma.
    e) Hepatoblastoma.

157. Pneumatosis cystoides intestinalis (Primary pneumatosis intestinalis) associated with:
    a) Chronic obstructive pulmonary disease.
    b) Bone marrow transplants.
    c) Cardiomyopathy.
    d) Necrotizing enterocolitis.
    e) Leukaemia.

158. Ascities in neoate is seen in the following:
    a) Prune belly syndrome.
    b) Neuroblastoma.
    c) Congenital biliary atresia.
    d) Erythroblastosis fetalis.
    e) Obstructive uropathy.

159. Causes of mesentreric vein thrombosis:
    a) Acute pancreatits.
    b) Liver cirrhosis.
    c) Malrotation of the bowel.
    d) Diverticulitis.
    e) Appendicitis.

160. The following are the venous causes of protein entropathy:
    a) Congestive heart failure.
    b) Constructive pericarditis.
    c) Tricuspid disease.
    d) Portal vein thrombosis.
    e) Splenic vein thrombosis.

161. The following are the lymphatic causes of protein losing enteropathy:
    a) Thoracic duct fistula.
    b) Whipple's disease.
    c) Reticulosis.
    d) Tropical sprue.
    e) Retroperitoneal fibrosis.

162. In coeliac axis compression syndrome:
    a) Post prandial pain and weight loss is a feature.
    b) Systolic abdominal murmur in all patients.
    c) Pain can be accentuated by deep expiration.

d) The narrowed area usually the end of the artery away from the origin of the celiac axis.
e) Post-stenotic dilation is a feature.

163. In ischemic colitis:
a) Occurs most commonly in pelvic colon.
b) A negative angiogram excluded this diagnosis.
c) Superficial ulceration is seen on barium enema examination.
d) There is gas in the bowel wall.
e) Spare the splenic flexure.

164. In Cushing's syndrome:
a) In adults, adenoma is a more common cause than bilateral adrenal hypoplasia.
b) In simple bilateral hyperplasia, ACTH is raised.
c) Is more common in men.
d) Hypercalcinuria occurs.
e) Associated with widening mediastrium.

165. In abdominal lymph glands the following are true:
a) Abdominoaortic group surround the aorta and inferior vena cava.
b) Visceral nodes drain adjacent organs including hepatic.
c) Hodgkin's lymphoma is much more common than non-Hodgkin's.
d) Conglomerate nodal masses are typical of lymphoma.
e) Low attenution within the enlarged nodes is usually represents necrosis on CT scan.

166. An increased incidence of peptic ulcer occurs in:
a) Hyperthyroidism.
b) Gout.
c) Cirrhosis of the liver.
d) Prolonged anti-coagulation therapy.
e) An insulin secreting tumour of the pancreas.

167. In caudate lobe of the liver:
a) Is also called quadrate lobe.
b) Is also called Riedel's lobe.
c) Is representing segment IV.

d) Is separated from the rest of the liver by the fissure of the ligamentum venosum anteriorly.
e) Supplied by branches of both right and left hepatic arteries and portal veins.

168. Omental cake usually seen in:
    a) Tuberculous peritonitis.
    b) Ovarian metastasis.
    c) Early testicular metastases.
    d) Gastric tumour metastases.
    e) Colonic cancer metastases.

169. The following are associated:
    a) Pedicle sign and metastasis.
    b) Trachea oesophageal fistula and Down syndrome.
    c) Malrotation of the bowel and cecal volvulus.
    d) Cecal volvulus and obstructed lesion of the left colon from diverticulitis.
    e) Internal hernia and tropical sprue.

170. In Feline oesphagus (oesophageal shiver):
    a) Permenant horizontal ridge throughout the upper oesophagus.
    b) Representing contraction mucosa.
    c) Seen in achalasia.
    d) Seen in association with hiatus hernia.
    e) Diagnosed only by endoscopy.

171. In imperforated anus:
    a) Associated with defect of the sacrum.
    b) Low defect of the rectum where the gab between the anal dimple and rectal stump is less than 1.5 cm.
    c) Fistula is common complication and indicates that the atresia is high.
    d) Radiological examination must be carried out immediately after birth.
    e) Infant held in inverted position for a few minutes to allow the air to completely distend the rectal segment.

172. Clinically significant protein loss may occur in:
    a) Radiation enteritis.
    b) Villous adenoma.

c) Whipple's disease.
d) Ulcerative colitis.
e) Intrathoracic stomach.

173. Which of the following statement are true:
    a) A gamma camera is better than at depth resolution than a melilinear scanner.
    b) Galcium 67 is excreted in bile.
    c) The common colloid particles used in lung scanning are under 300 m in diameter.
    d) Sialectasis occur in Sjogren's.
    e) Primary TB of the lung does not cavitate.

174. Which are true:
    a) Bile salts are secreted by the gallbladder.
    b) Bile salts are absorbed in the terminal ileum.
    c) Menetrier's disease is associated with renal calculi.
    d) Constructive pericarditis and protein losing entropathy.
    e) Enlarged temporal fossa associated with encephalitis.

175. Accessory pancreatic rests the following are true:
    a) Occur in fundus.
    b) Frequently undergo malignant change.
    c) May cause entero-enteric intussusception.
    d) May cause GI bleeding.
    e) May cause gastric outlet obstruction in neonate.

176. In Carcinoma of the oesophagus:
    a) Commonest site is middle third.
    b) There is an increased incidence in achalasia.
    c) There is increased incidence in obese subject.
    d) There is an increased incidence in cigarette smokers.
    e) Is retrosternal and mid mediastinal mass.

177. The following complications are common in Crohn's rather than ulcerative colitis:
    a) Fistula.
    b) Toxic dilation.
    c) Perforation.
    d) Carcinoma.
    e) Sclerosing Cholengitis.

178. The following radiological examination may be useful in the corresponding conditions:
   a) Barium swallow in hyperparathyroidism.
   b) Barium follow through the Sacroilitis.
   c) Barium enema in hydrocephalus infants.
   d) Angiogram in osteopoikilosis.
   e) CT scan of the skull with fibrous dysplasia of the vault.

179. Coeliac disease is associated with:
   a) Increased malignancy.
   b) Jaundice.
   c) Diverticulosis of the jejunum.
   d) Rapid transit time.
   e) Oedematous primary mucosal folds.

180. The following point to malignancy in a polyp:
   a) Greater than 1 cm in size.
   b) Irregular in outline.
   c) Multiple polyps.
   d) Increase in size.
   e) Pedunculated.

181. The following statements are true:
   a) Explosive diarrhoea occurs in Hirschsprung's disease.
   b) Double contrast barium enema is contraindicated in toxic mega colon.
   c) Streatorrhea is common in neurofibromatosis.
   d) The preparation of the patient in Hirschsprung's disease prior to barium enema is laxative for 2 days and washout enema.
   e) Water soluble contrast medium enema is contraindicated in the neonate.

182. In pancreas the following are true:
   a) The tail of the pancreas is entirely retroperitoneal.
   b) The typically measures 15–20 cm in length.
   c) The main pancreatic duct measures maximally 1.5 mm in the body.
   d) In most cases, the distal CBD and duct of Wirsung unite within the sphincter of Oddi.
   e) The duct of Santorini drains the posterior and inferior portions of the head via the minor papilla.

183. In pancreas the following are true:
   a) Fetal pancreatic lobulations are present in approximately 5% of people.
   b) Pancreas divisum is reported in approximately 9% of the population.
   c) If a cystic pancreatic lesion measures less than 3 cm, the likelihood of malignancy at that time is less than 3%.
   d) An anomalous pancreatic biliary junction is characterised by fusion of the pancreatic duct and CBD outside the sphincter of Oddi with formation of a long common channel that can increase the risk of acute recurrent pancreatitis.
   e) Autoimmune pancreatitis has been associated with other autoimmune disease, including Sjogren's syndrome, retroperitoneal fibrosis, primary Sclerosing cholangitis, rheumatoid arthritis, and inflammatory bowel disease.

184. In Intramural pseudodiverticulosis of the oesophagus:
   a) Candida organisms is predisposing factor.
   b) May found in patients with an otherwise normal oesophagus.
   c) On CT scan, thickening wall and irregularity of the lumen, mimicking esophageal carcinoma.
   d) Dysphagia lusoria can occur.
   e) Barium swallow is negative.

185. Abdominal enterolith seen in:
   a) Appendix.
   b) Meckel's diverticulum.
   c) Ileocecal valve.
   d) Diverticula.
   e) Pelvic veins.

186. In Meckel's diverticulum:
   a) Is a vestigial remnant of the omphalomesenteric duct.
   b) It is pseudodiverticulum.
   c) Adjacent to the ileocecal valve.
   d) Always contains hetrotopic tissue.
   e) Occur in 20% of the general population.

187. Gallbladder wall thickness seen in:
   a) Ascities.
   b) Acute cholecystitis.

c) Contracted after fatty meal.
d) Adenomyomatosis.
e) Haemobilia.

188. Drugs that produce esophageal ulceration and herpetic esophagitis.
    a) Tetracycline tablets.
    b) Aspirin tablets.
    c) Digoxine tablets.
    d) Potassium chloride tablets.
    e) Ascorbic acid tablets.

189. In Mirizzi syndrome:
    a) Gallstone impacted in the cystic duct or neck of the gallbladder.
    b) Intra hepatic bile ducts may become dilated.
    c) Obstructive jaundice is a feature.
    d) Endoscopic retrograde cholageiopancreatography (ERCP) is 95% accurate in complicated cases.
    e) Adenopathy may have a similar appearance.

190. The following are true small bowel Diverticulosis:
    a) Typically in the jejunum in location.
    b) Typically have narrow neck.
    c) Typically are asymptomatic.
    d) Lymphoma is recognised complication.
    e) Diverticulitis is recognised complication.

191. Intramural tracking in the colon on barium study seen in:
    a) Ascariasis.
    b) Angiodysplasia.
    c) Diverticulitis.
    d) Malignancy of the colon.
    e) Tuberculosis.

192. In backwash ileitis:
    a) Is a reflux ileitis.
    b) Polyps can develop in the terminal ileum.
    c) Yersinia species typically causes dilated-caliber terminal ileum.
    d) Crohn's typically causes narrowed-caliber terminal ileum.
    e) Ulcerative colitis typically causes normal-caliber terminal ileum.

193. In gallbladder polyps:
    a) Solitary could be papilloma.
    b) Multiple are likely cholesterol polyps.
    c) Mobile echogenic filling defects within the lumen on ultrasound.
    d) Can be move with changes in position.
    e) Multiple nodularity of the outer wall of the gallbladder is likely adenomyomatosis.

194. The following are true in spleenic laceration:
    a) The most commonly injured after blunt abdominal trauma.
    b) Diagnostic peritoneal lavage (DPL) accuracy is more than 90% in abdominal injury.
    c) Associated with fracture ribs in more than 90% of the cases.
    d) CT is the best modality when the patient is unstable.
    e) Evidence of active arterial extravasations diagnosed best by angiogram prior to surgery.

195. The following are true in varices of the oesophagus:
    a) Typically uphill direction due to liver disease.
    b) Typically downhill direction due to superior vena cava obstruction of azygos vein.
    c) Varices involve only the upper third if the superior vena cava blocked while the azygos vein is patent.
    d) Mediastinal adenopathy can produce uphill varices.
    e) Indwelling catheters of long duration may develop a thrombus of the superior vena cava and produce uphill varices.

196. The following are true in angiodysplasia of the colon (vascular ectasia):
    a) Is a congenital arterio venous malformation (AVM) of the descending colon.
    b) Predominantly affect young women and childhood.
    c) Associated with blood dyscrasia.
    d) Severe bleeding from the lower gastrointestinal tract is a feature.
    e) Diagnosed only by MR angiogram.

197. In Menetrier's disease of the stomach:
    a) Loss of normal thickness of the gastric folds.
    b) Associated with hypochloremia and hypoprotenemia.
    c) Is a recognised cause of protein-losing enteropathy.
    d) Patients often have pain, weight loss, vomiting, and diarrhoea.
    e) Can be diagnosed confidently by barium meal.

1. a. False   b. False   c. False   d. False   e. True

Epiploic appendagitis is an inflammatory/ischemic process involving an appendix epiploica of the colon. Maybe primary or secondary to adjacent pathology may be mimic to diverticulitis or appendicitis.
It is self limiting condition. Usually affects patients in their 2nd to 5th decades with a predilection for women and obese individuals.

Presented with pain and guarding distributed along the large bowel with variable frequency:
   Rectosigmoid junction 57%
   Ileocecal region 26%
   Ascending colon 9%

2. a. True   b. False   c. False   d. True   e. False

Killian-Jamieson Diverticulum
- Arises from cervical esophagus below cricopharyngeal muscle (about C5-C6) laterally
- Originates on the antero-lateral wall of cervical esophagus through a muscular gap (the Killian-Jamieson space) lateral to longitudinal muscle of the esophagus
- It is a pulsion, not a true diverticulum since it does not involve all layers of esophagus
- Usually smaller than a Zenker diverticulum
- Usually asymptomatic
- May produce reflux and aspiration
- Smooth-walled, contrast-containing pouch on barium swallow

Differential Diagnosis
- Zenker's diverticulum
  - o Arises above cricopharyngeal muscle in midline posteriorly
  - o Develops at anatomically weak posterior zone (Killian's dehiscence)

3. a. True   b. True   c. True   d. False   e. True

Choledochal cyst is a cystic dilation of the common bile duct.

Usually affect the supradoudenal portion and may also involve the hepatic and cystic ducts. Affected female more than males. Most cases present in the first two decades of life with pain, intermittent jaundice, and a palpable mass.

Types:
Type I – 80–90% secular or fusiform dilation of a portion or entire common bile duct with normal intrahepatic ducts.
Type II – isolated diverticulum protruding from CBD.
Type III or (Choledochocele) – arises from dilation duodenal portion of CBD or where pancreatic ducts meets.
Type IV – a. Multiple dilation of intra and extra hepatic biliary tree.
b. Multiple dilation involves only the extra hepatic bile ducts.
Type V – cystic dilation of the intra hepatic ducts.
Type VI – isolated cyst of the cystic duct very rare.

4. a. True   b. True   c. False   d. True   e. True

Macrocytic anaemia refers to a blood condition in which red blood cells are larger than normal. Several drugs can produce Macrocytic anaemia, e.g., Anticonvulsants agents, chemotherapeutic agents, Methotrexate, Cychlophosphamide, Sulfamethoxazole, Cladribine, Metformin, Zidovudine, and others such as alcoholism.

The uncomplicated hiatal hernia, stagnant loop, or Diverticulosis are not main direct causes. Crohn's disease is interfering with absorption.

5. a. True   b. False   c. False   d. True   e. False

Intramural hemorrhage can be fatal about 10% mortality rate. Barium enema should be avoided. Transcatheter embolization is the method of choice and intra arterial vasopressin infusion. There are several causes of intramural hemorrhage including vasculitis (Henoch-Schoniein Purpura). Coagulation defect including anticoagulation therapy, thrombocytopenia, disseminated intravascular coagulation. Also diasease with coagulation defect such as leukemia, multiple myeloma, hemophilia, lymphoma, metastatic carcinoma. Ischemia and trauma are also causes.

Radiography appears as stacked coin and picket fence of mucosal folds, it may shows as thumb printing shape due to focal accumulation of hematoma in bowel wall.

6.   a. True   b. True   c. False   d. True   e. True

Polydipsia – chronic excessive thirst and fluid intake. May be due to diabetes, decreased blood volume as occurs during major haemorrhage or other conditions that create a water deficit. It can be symptom of anti-cholinergic poisoning. Antipsychotics can have side effects such as dry mouth, seen also in hyperaldoteronism mental illness such as schizophrenia.

7.   a. True   b. True   c. False   d. False   e. False

Crohn's disease (regional enteritis) is chronic granulomatous condition which may affect any part of the gut, commonly the terminal ileum. Several separate of the area of the disease (skip lesions) may be present. The bowel wall is thickened, congested, and rigid, it's lumen usually narrowed and ulcerated, involve the rectum in about 30% of the cases. Associated with gallstone, fistula, and sinuses are common while toxic mega colon is rare so as perforation and malignant changes.

8.   a. False   b. True   c. True   d. False   e. False

Peptic ulceration occurs in those parts of the alimentary canal, which are bathed in the acid/peptin secretions. However, it may be associated with trauma or burns. It may be seen as result of ingestion of drugs, e.g., aspirin, Butazolin, or steroids, etc. Healed ulcer may cause fibrosis giving rise to pyloric stenosis if the ulcer is situated to pyloric canal, or less frequently to an hour-glass deformity of the stomach if the ulcer lies in the body of the stomach. Best diagnosed by fibro optic endoscopy, it may be multiple, it may be acute or chronic, it may be small or large, benign or malignant. Gastric ulcer can perforate, penetrate, bleed, and deform the stomach.

9. a. True   b. False   c. False   d. True   e. True

The retropharyngeal space in an infant or child can be seen in enlarged adenoids or tonsils, retropharyngeal abscess or cellulitis, trauma (haematoma or spine fracture), cretinism (my edema), cystic hygroma (lymphnagioma), foreign body, haemangioma, retropharyngeal goiter, spinal lesion, e.g., tuberculosis or metastasis. Truamatic pseudodiverticulum of pharynx (from finger in infant's mouth during delivery) tumours, e.g., plexiform neurofibroma, lymphoma, or angiofibroma.

10. a. True   b. True   c. False   d. True   e. True

Malrotation of bowel is abnormal positioning gut secondary to narrow mesenteric attachment as a result of arrest in the embryonic development of gut rotation with abnormal fixation of mesentery. The mesentery is short. It is associated with asplenia and midabdominal location of the liver. May presents with intestinal obstruction. The duodenal-jejunal flexure takes Z-shape configuration. It associated with large bowel volvulus. Can be associated also with exomphalos, prune belly syndrome, pseudo obstruction of the urinary tract.

11. a. False   b. True   c. True   d. True   e. False

Congenital Diaphragmatic Hernia
Herniation of abdominal contents into the chest typically via a posterior defect in the diaphragm (Bochdalek hernia). Classical imaging appearance, bubble-like lucencies that appear like bowel within the chest, mediastinal shift, compressed lung. Presented at birth with severe respiratory distress, hernia may contain stomach (intra thoracic stomach), small bowel, colon, and liver, more common on the left side than right.

12. a. True   b. False   c. True   d. True   e. True

Protein-Losing Disorders of the Gastrointestinal Tract
Protein is continually entering the lumen of the gut in the form of shed mucosal cells, lymph, and other secretion. Normally most of it absorbed. In a wide variety of conditions, there may be excessive loss of protein so that the protein balance becomes negative. Patients presents with oedema.

Some cuases:
1. Lymphatic, e.g., Whipple's disease, reticulosis, thoracic ducts obstruction.
2. Venous, e.g., congestive heart failure, constrictive pericarditis, thrombosis, etc.
3. Ulceration, e.g., carcinoma of the stomach or colon, villous adenoma.
4. Unknown, e.g., Menetrier's disease, gluten induces enteropathy, eosinophilic enteropathy.

13. a. True   b. True   c. True   d. False   e. True

Acute appendicitis is due to obstruction of appendicular lumen by lymphoid hyperplasia 60% or fecolith 33%, foreign bodies 4%, stricture, tumour parasite, Crohn's disease 25%.

80% clinical accuracy in male, crampy pain migrates into right lower quadrant. Pain over appendix (McBurney sign).

The plain abdominal film may help in diagnosis, may shows laminated calcified appendicolith in right lower quadrant. Air/fluid level on erect film may see a gas loculation or intraluminal gas, distortion of Psoas margin and flank strips. Scoliosis due to muscle irritation.

14. a. False   b. True   c. True   d. True   e. False

Meconium ileus – inspissations of the meconium in the large bowel results in obstruction of the small bowel, usually by a plug of meconium in the terminal ileum. Distended loops of small bowel are present without fluid levels.

Gastrografin enema has been used as a curative procedure because of the hyperosmolarity softens the meconium and allows the obstruction to be relieved. However gastrografin enema may cause hypovolemia and dehydration of the infant. Necrosis of the mucosal colon may happen in hypertonic solution in prolong procedure. The plain abdomen may also show tiny calcification within the pancreatic region in the mid upper abdomen as well as in the peripheries within the peritoneum.

Pneomoperitonium is common complication due to rupture of the bowel loops.

15. a. False   b. True   c. True   d. True   e. False

Glucagon – peptid hormone secreted by the pancreas. Its affect is opposite that of insulin.

Therapeutic value of glucagon in hydrostatic reduction of ileocolic intussusceptions and other condition.

16. a. True   b. True   c. False   d. True   e. True

Ascites in neonates denaotes an intraperitoneal accumulation of fluid during prenatal life or shortly after birth.

Extravasation of urine from the ruptured kidneys (urinoma) can give to ascites. Prune belly syndrome that occurs in boy with thin or lax abdominal wall, tortuous, dilated ureters, and cytochidism.

17. a. True   b. True   c. True   d. False   e. False

Gastric polyps – most common benign gastric tumour. Associated with hyperacidity and ulcers, chronic atrophic gastritis, and gastric carcinoma.
- A. Hyperplastic polyp (inflammatory polyp) (75–90%).
- B. Adenomatous polyp (10–20%). Associated with Gardner's syndrome, juvenile polyposis, and Cronkhite-Canada syndrome and occurs more commonly in antrum.
- C. Hamartomatous polyp (rare). Associated with Peutz-Jeghers syndrome. Usually < 2 cm in diameter.
- D. Retention polyp (rare). Dilated cystic glands. Associated with Cronkhite-Canada syndrome.
- E. Villous polyp.

18. a. False   b. True   c. False   d. True   e. True

Porcelain Gallbladder
Calcification of all or part of the gallbladder wall.
- Less than 1% cholecystectomy patients. F:M – 5:1, flakes of dystrophic calcium within chronically inflamed and fibrotic muscular wall. Wall is thickened and gallbladder is contracted.

- Associated with gallstones in 90%. Cystic duct is always obstructed. 80% of patients with carcinoma of gallbladder have stones.
- Patients are usually asymptomatic.

Imaging Findings
- On conventional radiographs or CT, curvilinear calcifications in segment of the wall or entire wall. CT is more sensitive than conventional radiographs. Thickness of calcification may vary.
- On ultrasound, highly echogenic, shadowing, curvilinear structure in gallbladder fossa.
- Echogenic gallbladder wall with little acoustic shadowing.
- Large gallstone with peripheral calcification may give imaging pit fall.
- Because of its high association with carcinoma of the gallbladder, a cholycystectomy is usually performed.
- 20–30% develops carcinoma of gallbladder.

19. a. False   b. True   c. True   d. True   e. False

Diabetes Mellitus
Multisystem disorder – macrovascular and microvascular disease, neuropathy, increase susceptibility to infection, e.g., renal and perineal abscesses, emphysematous, pyelonephritis, emphysematous cystitis, fungal infection, candida, aspergillus, xanthogranulomatous pyelonephritis, Fournier gangrene.

The palin abdomen x-ray shows calcification of vas deferens in older diabetic patient and also shows vascular calcification.

20. a. False   b. True   c. True   d. True   e. False

Air in the biliary tree seen in association with fistula, e.g., choledochoenteric, choledochodoudenal, or cholecystodoudenal. It may occur in post choledochojejusnostomy or other iatrogenic cause, e.g., sphincterotomy.

In Miirizzi syndrome there is a biliary obstruction by a gallbladder stone impacted in the cystic duct induces cholangitis or erodes into the common duct to cause obstructive jaundice. The width of the common bile duct normally < 7 mm and it is dilated when the obstruction between the ampulla of vater below the level of the cystic duct.

Parasitic cause of obstructive jaundice can be due to ascaris or clonorchis.

Klatkin's tumour is occurs at the confluence of dilated right and left hepatic ducts.

21. a. False   b. False   c. False   d. False   e. True

The superior mesenteric artery syndrome is a compression of the third, transverse portion of the duodenum.

The angle between SMA and aorta is 45–65 degrees and it reduced to 10–20 in this position.

The compression is worse when the patient is in the supine position and not relieved in the prone position.

The vertical linear compression defect is seen in the third part of duodenum.

The gross dilation of the duodenum proximal to the level of compression and the distal portion is collapsed.

22. a. False   b. True   c. True   d. True   e. True

23. a. True   b. True   c. True   d. True   e. False

24. a. True   b. True   c. True   d. True   e. False

25. a. True   b. True   c. True   d. False   e. True

26. a. True   b. True   c. True   d) True   e. False

27. a. False   b. True   c. True   d. False   e. False

28. a. True   b. True   c. True   d. True   e. False

29. a. True   b. True   c. True   d. False   e. True

30. a. True   b. False   c. True   d. True   e. True

31. a. True   b. False   c. True   d. True   e. True

32.	a. True	b. True	c. True	d. True	e. False
33.	a. False	b. True	c. True	d. True	e. False
34.	a. False	b. True	c. True	d. True	e. False
35.	a. False	b. True	c. True	d. False	e. True
36.	a. True	b. True	c. True	d. False	e. True
37.	a. False	b. True	c. True	d. False	e. True
38.	a. False	b. True	c. False	d. True	e. False
39.	a. True	b. True	c. False	d. True	e. True
40.	a. True	b. True	c. True	d. True	e. False
41.	a. False	b. True	c. True	d. True	e. False
42.	a. False	b. True	c. True	d. True	e. True
43.	a. True	b. True	c. True	d. True	e. False
44.	a. True	b. False	c. False	d. False	e. True
45.	a. True	b. True	c. True	d. False	e. False
46.	a. True	b. True	c. True	d. False	e. True
47.	a. False	b. False	c. False	d. True	e. True
48.	a. True	b. True	c. True	d. True. False	
49.	a. True	b. True	c. False	d. True	e. True
50.	a. True	b. True	c. False	d. True	e. True
51.	a. True	b. True	c. True	d. True	e. False
52.	a. True	b. True	c. False	d. False	e. False

53. a. True   b. True   c. True   d. True   e. False

54. a. True   b. True   c. True   d. False   e. True

55. a. True   b. False   c. True   d. False   e. True

56. a. False   b. True   c. True   d. True   e. True

57. a. False   b. False   c. True   d. True   e. False

58. a. False   b. False   c. True   d. False   e. True

59. a. True   b. True   c. True   d. False   e. False

60. a. False   b. True   c. False   d. True   e. True

61. a. False   b. True   c. True   d. True   e. True

62. a. False   b. True   c. True   d. True   e. True

63. a. True   b. False   c. True   d. True   e. False

Also seen in Zollinger-Ellision syndrome, sprue chagas disease, superior mesenteric artery syndrome, drugs, e.g., probanthine, atropine, morphine; ileus, scleroderma, congenital atresia, stenosis, annular pancreas, etc.

64. a. True   b. True   c. False   d. True   e. False

65. a. True   b. True   c. True   d. True   e. False

66. a. False   b. False   c. False   d. True   e. True

67. a. True   b. False   c. True   d. True   e. False

68. a. True   b. False   c. True   d. True   e. True

69. a. True   b. True   c. False   d. True   e. True

70. a. False   b. False   c. False   d. True   e. False

Chilaiditi's Sign/Syndrome
Hepatodiaphragmatic interposition of the intestine
- Pronounced 'Ky-La-Ditty'.
- Refers to the usually asymptomatic interposition of the bowel (usually hepatic flexure of the colon) between the liver and the (right) hemidiaphragm.
- Almost always in adult males.

Clinical Finding:
The 'symptume' may involve abdominal pain, constipation, vomiting, respiratory distress, and anorexia.

Chilaiditi's syndrome is important because it can simulate Pneumoperitonium; look for the presence of haustral folds which can establish the air beneath the diaphragm is contained within large bowel.

71. a. True   b. True   c. True   d. True   e. False

72. a. True   b. False   c. True   d. True   e. False

73. a. True   b. True   c. True   d. False   e. True

Hyperamylasemia
Raised serum amylase and lipase levels are observed in several abdominal diseases, pancreatitis, biliary tract disease, perforated gastroduodenal ulcer, and acute appendicitis.

Ectopic pregnancy, salivary gland infection, some medication that could heighten the amount of amylase in the blood includes aspirin, birth control pills, cholinergic medications, methyldopa, opiates (codeine, meperidine, morphine).

74. a. True   b. True   c. True   d. False   e. True

Paralytic Ileus
Acute obstructive small bowel distention occurs in:
1. Electrolyte imbalance (e.g., hypokalemia, hypochloremia, calcium, and magnesium abnormalities)
2. Loclaized sentinel loop (e.g., hepatic flexure in acute cholcystitis, terminal ileum in appendicitis, transverse colon or jejunum in acute pancreatitis, descending colon in diverticulitis)

3. Others – shock septicemia, renal calculus, post operative, adrenal insufficiency pophyria, diabetic acidosis, insulin shock, sickle cell crisis, aerophagia, acute glomerulonephritis, etc.

75. a. True   b. False   c. True   d. True   e. True

Henoch-Schonlein Pupura (Anaphylactoid Purpura/Purpura rheumatic) is a disease of skin and other organs affecting the small vessels (vasculitis), affected the joints, gastrointestinal tract, and urinary tract (glomerulonephritis).

Erosive arthropathy seen in gout, pseudogout syndrome, hemochromatosis, alkaptonuria, acromegaly, and others.

76. a. True   b. True   c. False   d. True   e. False

Pernicious anaemia caused by luck of intrinsic factor or other causes such as infections, surgery, medicine or diet; e.g., malabsorption in the small bowel, celiac disease, Crohn's disease, inflammatory bowel diseases, antibiotic, diabetes, and seizure medication.

Surgical removal of part or all small bowel.

Tapeworm infestation.

77. a. True   b. True   c. False   d. False   e. False

Intussusception
Forward peristalsis results invagination of more proximal bowel (the intussusception) into lumen of more distal bowel (the intussuscepiens) in a telescope-like manner. 90% idiopathic, 2% due to lymphoid hyperplasia. Most common between 3 months and 12 months of age.

Rarely in older children other causes should be considered including lymphoma, Henoch-Schonlein purpura, duplication, Meckle diverticulum.

Image guided pressure reduction, treatment of choice with high success rate. Pucity of RLQ gas on plain abdomen also non-visualisation of air-filled cecum. Signs of small bowel obstruction (air fluid levels in erect film).

On ultrasound, pseudo-kidney appearance on longitudinal images.

On CT scan, colonic mass with alternating rings of high and low attenuation. May not be located in RLQ of intussusception has progressed distal.

78. a. False   b. False   c. False   d. True   e. False

Necrotizing Enterocolitis (NEC)
Idiopathic enterocolitis that is most likely related to some combination of infection and ischemia.

Disease of premature infants, typically in the intensive care unit. Classic appearance pneumatosis in right lower quadrant affected the ileum and ascending colon.

Strictures is recognised complication and portal venous gas, Pneumoperitonium, ascites, football sign (outline of falciform ligament). Rigler's sign (in visualisation of both sides of bowel walls).

79. a. False   b. True   c. False   d. True   e. False

Cushing's Syndrome
- Excessive production of glucocorticoids.
- Approximately 70% of cases are due to adrenal hyperplasia resulting from Adrenocortropic Hormone (ACTH).
- About 20% are due to adrenal adenoma, 10% due to adrenal carcinoma.
- About 80% of all patients are women, most commonly age 20 to 40 years.
- Increase fat deposition in the subcutaneous tissues, abdomen, and liver.
- May be iatrogenic (increased administration of corticosteroids).
- May be associated with bronchial bronchial carcinoma, hypercalcemia, islet cell tumour of pancreas.
- Widening of mediastinum on postero anterior view of the chest radiograph may be present.

80. a. True   b. True   c. True   d. True   e. False

Oesophagitis in Infancy
- Inflammation of the oesophagus often caused by gastroesophageal reflux. A response of body tissue to injury or irritation characterised by and swelling and redness and heat. Ulcer may develop and symptoms can be cured medically including haematemesis.
- There is no relation between sideropenic web and this condition.
- Cricopharyngeal web (Paterson-Brown Kelly syndrome) or called Plummer-Vinson syndrome occurs in middle aged females associated with iron deficiency anaemia and presented with dysphagia. The location of the web in the post-cricoid region.

81. a. False   b. True   c. True   d. False   e. False

Megacolon of an infant or child very much dilated colon including Hirschsprung's disease (colonic aganglionosis). Is functional obstruction of the distal colon secondary to lack of innervations ganglion cells.

Some other causes of megacolon including functional psychogenic, idiopathic, imperforated anus, toxic mega colon, anal fissure, duplication, neurogenic (e.g., meningmyelocele, other spinal abnormalities), pelvic tumour (e.g., teratoma), and post rectal stricture.

Turcot syndrome is multiple adenomatous polyps with risk of colorectal cancer and brain tumour (medulloblastoma).

82. a. True   b. True   c. True   d. False   e. True

The following are associated with:
a) Erythema nodosum is an acute inflammatory skin disease marked by ender red nodules, usually on the skins due to exudation of blood and serum. It may be due to leprosy or other inflammatory condition, administration of drugs or toxic substance.
b) Gorln syndrome (a navoid basal carcinoma syndrome) is basal naevus syndrome which associated with odontogenic cysts in the jaw, rib anomalies, broad forehead.
c) Albright syndrome is fibrous dysplasia, skin pigmentation, precious puberty (almost exclusively in female).
d) Can involve the liver, may be multiple, but the liver is not obviously enlarged clinically.

83. a. True   b. True   c. False   d. True   e. True

Coeliac Disease
- Adult coeliac disease or gluten-induced enteropathy.
- Partial or subtotal villous atrophy.
- There is dilatation of the jejunum results in the secondary folds being smooth out, revealing the primary transverse folds (the valvulae coniventes).
- Patients are with hypokalemia. Lymphoma is a common complication. Jaundice may be present transit time of the intestinal content is rapid.

84. a. False   b. True   c. True   d. False   e. True

Cecal Volvulus
- Volvulus is 3rd most common cause of colonic obstruction. Following obstructing carcinoma and inflammatory stricture.
- Two most common forms are cecal and sigmoid.
- Cecal volvulus can be associated with malrotation of the colon. Abnormality long mesentery of cecum and ascending colon leads to mobility of right colon predisposing to volvulus. Other factors must be at play, though, since 10% of population has such a long mesentery yet few develop cecal volvulus. Cecal volvulus has been associated with obstructing lesions of the left colon from carcinoma or diverticulitis.
- Ascending colo twists on its longitudinal axis from 180° to 360° and rotates cecum upward and to left of midline.
- Age peak: 20–40 years; M > F.
- Patients present most often with an acute abdomen. Colicky abdominal pain of sudden onset.
- Most cases of cecal volvulus reportedly occur in patients while they are asleep with normal side to side movement during sleep possibly resulting in displacement of the right colon to an abnormal location.
- Diagnosis is usually by plain film appearance.

Imaging Findings
- Markedly dilated cecum. 'Kidney-shaped' distended cecum. Usually positioned in LUQ or to the left midline.
- Most obstructions are complete so there is little gas in the rest of the colon.

- If barium enema is done, tapered and of barium column points toward torsion. Beak configuration to end of barium column.
- About 10–33% of cecal volvuli are cecal bascules. Cecum does not rotate around its luminal axis. Consistent feature of cecal bascule in presence of a constricting band across the ascending colon, the origin of which is not certain. Cecum folds anteromedial to the ascending colon produces a flap-valve occlusion at the site of flexion. Occurs in a transverse plane and is associated with marked distention of the cecum. Often displaced into the centre of the abdomen.
- Findings: distended air-filled cecum is located more centrally.

85. a. True   b. True   c. True   d. True   e. False

Polypoid lesions of the colon historically classified as adenomatous, villous adenoma, juvenile polyps, Pentz-Jegher's polyp, post-inflammatory polyps.

The benign polyp is less than 10 mm in size. Pedunculated polyp with long stalk is likely benign while sessile polyp with diameter of base greater than height is likely malignant. Single smooth surface of the polyp is usually benign.

Colon contour of irregular wall is malignant.

86. a. False   b. True   c. False   d. True   e. True

Gastric Diverticulum

General Considerations
- Congenital, contain all layers usually on the posterior wall of the stomach at the cardia.
- May be intramural which projects into muscular layer usually on the greater curvature of the antrum however it may contains mucosa and submucosa without muscularis propia.
- Often near the esophagogastric junction while the acquired diverticula may be associated with peptic ulcer disease, bowel obstruction, cancer, and gastric surgery.
- Usually asymptomatic often found incidentally on imaging.
- May rarely be symptomatic and then, usually when diverticulum is in the prepyloric region.

- Symptoms may include epigastric pain, lower chest pain, abdominal pain, dyspepsia, bleeding, and nonbilious emesis.

Imaging Findings
- Barium study – well-circumscribed, barium or air-containing, rounded outpouching with an air-fluid level if the patient is upright.
- Endoscopy – diverticulum with a well-defined opening.
- Computed Tomography – outpouching that distorts the normal contour of the stomach.

Complications
- Haemorrhage, ulceration, perforation, and torsion.
- May be associated with an increase risk of malignancy.

87. a. True   b. True   c. True   d. True   e. False

Adrenal Calcification

General Considerations
- Haemorrhage is the most common cause.
- Most (90%) of adrenal tissue must be destroyed for adrenal insufficiency.
- Adrenal haemorrhage is prognostically important because it may signify severe stress or unsuspected coagulopathy.
- Causes are haemorrhage, TB, or Histoplasmosis, almost always unilateral neuroblastoma, pheochromocytoma may be bilateral or ectopic, Addison's disease after the cortex and Wolman's disease.

Imaging Findings
- CT is the study of choice in adults
  - Adrenal haemorrhage and haemorrhagic adrenal rumors may appear similar.
  - Follow-up in 4 weeks to resolution for haemorrhage, tumours will not resolve.
  - Acute haemorrhage is hyperdense.
  - Associated with inflammatory stranding.
  - Adrenal is usually enlarged.
  - Bronchogenic carcinoma metastatic to the adrenals is the most common cause of an enlarged and haemorrhagic adrenal malignancy.
- Ultrasound (US) is the modality of choice in neonates.

- • Sensitive to enlargement.
- • Glands may be large and hyperechoic early and hyperechoic centrally later.
- MRI may be useful is evaluating the stage of haemorrhage.
- On conventional radiography, adrenal calcifications will usually be bilateral and amorphous. Located in the region of the adrenals, adjacent to the spine.
- Calcification may be seen within weeks of the haemorrhage.

88. a. True   b. True   c. False   d. False   e. True

Carcinoma of the Colon
Some risk factors – polyps, family history of benign or malignant colon tumours, chronic ulcerative colitis, Crohn's disease, prior pelvic radiation, in women who have carcinoma of breast or uterus, retinitis pigmentosa, Gardener's syndrome, and adenocarcinomas make up the vast majority.

Clinical – peak age 50–60 years, weight loss, blood in stool, loss of appetite, change in bowel habits.

Common location – recto sigmoid region, more common in left colon with chronic ulcerative colitis.

Imaging findings – 90–95% rate of detection by BE double contrast as polypoid filling defect or annular constricting = apple-core lesion; Scirrhous ca. – rare infiltrating type which gives lead-pipe appearance seen especially in ulcerative colitis.

Metastases – liver (25%), retroperitoneal and mesenteric nodes (15%), hydronephrosis (13%), adrenal (10%) and ascites. Complications: obstruction – may be retrograde but not antegrade more likely to be left-sided than right-sided, perforation, intussusception, pneumatosis intestinalis.

89. a. True   b. False   c. False   d. True   e. False

The concentration of barium used for the different examinations for GI tract are:
- Barium swallow and meal 250% weight/volume.
- For follow through and small bowel enema is 60%.
- For large bowel barium enema is about 100% weight/volume.

90. a. True   b. False   c. True   d. False   e. True

Esophageal atresia (EA) and Tracheoesophageal Fistula

Esophageal atresia with fistulous connection to distal pouch is more common than esophageal atresia alone or tracheoesophageal fistula without esophageal atresia (H-type fistula).
- Esophageal atresia with fistula about 80%.
- Esophageal atresia with no fistula about 9%.
- No esophageal atresia only bronchoesophageal fistula (H-shape) is about 6%.

Increased incidence of tracheoesophageal fistula with Down syndrome and prematurity. May be associated with duodenal atresia or stenosis, imperforated anus, 13 pairs of ribs may be present, number of lumbar vertebra may be 6.

VACTERL represent V = vertebral, A = anal atresia, C = cardiac anomalies, TE = tracheoesophageal fistula or atresia, R = renal agenesis and dysplasia, limb defects.

The symptoms in general include choking, regurgitation, aspiration and respiratory distress.

The H-type may diagnosed at late childhood. Prenatal ultrasound can suggest diagnosis as early as 24 weeks because polyhydramnious. Aspiration pneumonia is common with esophageal atresia without fistula there will be no air enters GI tract.

91. a. True   b. True   c. True   d. False   e. False

Carcinoid Tumour of the Small Bowel
Potentially malignant, neuroendocrine tumour of primitive stem cells in gut wall which have hormone-secreting potential – arise from enterochromaffin cells of Kulchitsky. ~50% of carcinoids occur in appendix; ~33% occur in small bowel. Most common primary tumour of the small bowel. Most common presentation is episodic abdominal pain, usually associated with liver metastasis. Usually performed once biochemical diagnosis confirmed, typically by elevated 24-hour excretion of 5-HIAA.

Abdominal CT with intravenous and oral contrast – visualisation of primary tumour; lymph node enlargement—mesenteric, para-aortic or retroperitoneal; radiating linear strands around soft tissue mass due to fibrosis ("spoke-wheel" pattern); may contain calcification; bowel wall thickening of adjacent bowel loops; liver metastases—often multiple, frequently associated with carcinoid syndrome; ischemia or obstruction due to fibrosis may be present; carcinoid tumour cells almost always contain somatostatin receptors, and show increased uptake on scan; more sensitive than MIGB scans.

MRI with gadolinium – useful for detection of metastases; low T1 and high T2; enhance peripherally in arterial phase and hypointense during venous phase.

Complications – carcinoid syndrome, carcinoid crisis, carcinoid heart disease, intussusception associated with scleroderma.

92. a. False   b. True   c. True   d. False   e. True

Emphysematous Cholecystitis

General Considerations
- Acute infection of gallbladder caused by gas-forming organism. In about 1/3 = clostridium perfringens. Also E. coli and Klebsiella.
- Rare – only 1% of all cases of acute cholecyatitis.
- Occurs more often in men. As opposed to gallbladder disease in general which occurs more often in women.
- Most are elderly patients (> 60) with diabetes.
- Vascular compromise of the cystic artery may play a role in the etiology. Gallstones may be associated with the disease but are not thought to cause it.
- Gas may occur in the wall and/or the lumen. May spread to pericholecystic tissue. Rarely, gas may escape into the bile ducts. This is rare since cystic duct is usually occluded in cholecystitis.

Clinical Findings
- As with cholecystitis, right upper quadrant (RUQ) pain and tenderness.
- Leukocytes.
- Jaundice is rare.

Imaging Findings
- Conventional radiography
  - May show air in the wall or lumen of the gallbladder.
  - Air-filled levels in the gallbladder will only be seen with images obtained with a horizontal beam, not on supine radiographs.
  - Gas may spread to the pericholecystic tissue.
  - These findings, if present on the conventional radiograph, usually herald a poor outcome from late-stage disease.

- Ultrasound findings
  - Indistinct shadowing emanating from wall or lumen of gallbladder.
  - 'Ring-down effect' or 'come tail' from shadowing from air in gallbladder lumen.

- CT findings of cholecystitis
  - Air in gallbladder wall is diagnostic of this disease.
  - Most common signs of non-emphysematous cholecystitis are gallbladder wall thickening > 3 mm
  - Cholelithiasis.
  - Increased density of bile (>20 H).
  - Loss of clear definition of gallbladder wall.
  - Pericholecytic fluid such as a halo of edema.

93. a. True   b. False   c. False   d. False   e. False

Hodgkin's Disease
- Hodgkin's – disease of T cells.
- Bimodal peaks at age 25–30 years and 75–80 years.
- Represent 40% of lymphoma.
- Associated with generalised pruritis night sweats, weight loss, alcohol-induced pain, and painless lymphadenopathy.

94. a. False   b. True   c. True   d. True   e. True

Hepatic Haemangioma
- A common benign liver lesion up of vascular channels with slowly circulating blood. Most are clinically silent.
- Kasaback-Merritt syndrome is the association of a large haemangioma and thrombocytopenia.

- On ultrasound, the majority uniformly hyperechoic and unchange in size on follow up, some may be heterogenous owing to scaring fibrosis, or haemorrhage.
- On CT scan with 3-phase, which comprises a precontrast series, an arterial phase series and a portal phase. Occasionally delayed series are required.
- Haemangioma are low density on precontrast imaging.
- On every post contrast there is no nodular peripheral enhancement.
- Delay imaging shows filling in from the pherphery inwards. This result in complete 'in-fill' in three-quarters of haemangiomas. Large haemangiomas are more likely not to fill in completely owing to increased incidence of central scarring.
- Small < 1 cm may not demonstrate classical peripheral, nodular enhancement, being seen as a homogenous enhancing lesion on early phase imaging.
- The differential includes hypervascular metastases but these wash out on delayed imaging and are then hypodense caompared with normal hepatic parenchyma.
- Haemagiomas remain hyperdense on delayed images.

95. a. True   b. True   c. False   d. False   e. True

Infantile Hypertrophic Pyloric Stenosis
- Idiopathic thickening of pyloric muscle in infancy, which creates progressive gastric outlet obstruction.
- Typically 2- to 4-week-old infants with worsening projectile vomiting. Palpable olive-shaped mass.
- Male more than female.
- On ultrasound, thickening of the pylorus > 3 mm, pyloric channel length > 16 mm, pyloric diameter > 15 mm.
- On fluoroscopy, overdistended stomach, caterpillar stomach, exaggerated gastric motility.
- Tram track or string sign of barium within narrowed channel.

96. a. True   b. True   c. True   d. False   e. False

Ileal Atresia
Congenital obstruction of ileum secondary to in utero ischemia. Unlike duodenal atresia jejuno ileal atresia associated with in utero ischemic event.

Classic imaging appearance, distal bowel obstruction with bulbus bowel segment. Radiologically distal bowel obstruction with dilated loops proximal to atresia with fluid-filled, may appear soft tissue mass, contrast enema findings microcolon, colon may contain some meconium calcification when meconium peritonitis present.

Should be differentiated from the:
    a.   Meconium ileus
    b.   Meconium plug syndrome (small left colon syndrome)
    c.   Hirschsprung's disease

Treated surgically with potential complications of short gut syndrome, dismotility contrast study with dilute ionic-water soluble agents.

97.   a. True   b. False   c. True   d. True   e. True

Hepatoblastoma is most common hepatic malignancy in infants and children, more in boys.

Positive serum alpha-fetaprotein, predisposing condition, Beck-Wiedemann syndrome, biliary atresia.

On ultrasound, mass typically hypervascular on doppler sonography.

Heterogenous echogenicity from haemorrhage of necrosis.

C.T. shows mass typically well-defined and heterogeneous, usually calcified tend to displace or invade adjacent hepatic structure.

98.   a. True   b. True   c. False   d. False   e. False

Cirrhosis chronic liver disease characterised by diffuse parenchymal necrosis, regeneration and scarring with abnormal reconstruction of preexisting lobular architecture.

Etiology:
    A.   Toxic
            1.   Alcohol live disease in 75%
            2.   Drug-induced (prolonged Methotrexate, oxyphenisatin, alpha-methyldopa, nitrofurantoin, isoniazid)
            3.   Iron overload (hemochromatosis, hemosiderosis)

- B. Inflammation
    1. Viral hepatitis
    2. Schistosomiasis
- C. C. Biliary Obstruction
    1. Cystic fibrosis
    2. Inflammatory bowel disease
    3. Primary biliary cirrhosis
    4. Obstructive infantile cholangiopathy
- D. D. Vascular
    1. Prolonged CHF = cardiac cirrhosis
    2. Hepatic venoocclusis disease (Budd-Chiari syndrome)
- E. Nutritional
    1. Intestinal bypass
    2. Severe steatosis
    3. Abetalipoproteinemia
- F. Hereditary
1. Wilson disease
2. Alpha-1 antitrypsin deficiency
3. Juvenile polycystic kidney diasease
4. Galactosemia
5. Type IV glycogen storage disease
6. Hereditary fructose intolerance
7. Tyrosinemia
8. Hereditary tetany
9. Osler-Weber-Rendu syndrome
10. Familial cirrhosis
- G. Idiopathic/cryptogenic

99. a. True   b. True   c. False   d. False   e. True

Pneumoperitonium
- Presence of air or gas in the peritoneal cavity as result of disease or iatrogenic trauma. Causes include perforated hallow viscus, inflammation, and ileus. Minimal air can be seen on left lateral decubitus view of the abdomen. However CT scan is the best modality.
- Rigler's sign is ment to the ability to see both sides of the bowel wall because there is gas on both sides. Reabsorb air in thick patients take longer perhaps because overweight patient have a fatty omentum.

100. a. False   b. False   c. False   d. True   e. True

Whipple's disesase is caused by Trapheryma, whipelli, a gram positive organism. It is characterised by presence of PAS positive, material in the foamy macrophages in the submucosa of small bowel.

Arthritis precedes intestinal disease in 10%. Generalised lymphadenopathy is seen in 50%.

It is eight time common in males.

101. a. True   b. True   c. True   d. False   e. False

Thickened, irregular folds in small bowel are seen in:
- May be due to infection, e.g., TB, giardiasis, strongyloidosis.
- Or Inflammatory, e.g., Crohn's disease, Zollinger-Ellison syndrome.
- Infiltrative, e.g., amyloidosis eosinophic entiritis, Whipple's disease, mastocytosis.

102. a. True   b. True   c. True   d. True   e. False

Chronic intestinal pseudo obstruction can be primary or secondary pseudo-obstruction include side to side anastomosis bypassed bowel, pouches, dermatomyoositis, polymyositis, amyloidosis, Chagas disease, diabetes, tricyclic antidepression, and NASID.

103. a. False   b. True   c. True   d. True   e. True

Mechanical Intestinal Obstruction in Children
  A. High obstruction (Proximal to mid ileum) bilious vomiting (after feeding) or abdominal distention, few dilated bowel loops.
  B. Low obstruction (Distal ileum/colon) requires contrast enema examination to diagnose microcolon, position of cecum.
  - Abdominal distention plus vomiting.
  - Failure to pass meconium.
  - Many dilated intestinal loops.
  - Some of the common cause of intestinal obstruction in children including volvulus, atresia bands, annular pancreas, duplication, diverticulum, and others.

The abdominal plain film shows double bubble sign (air-fluid levels) in the stomach and 50–60% sensitive. Candy cone appearance in erect film position > 3 cm distended small bowel loops, > 3 cm gas fluid levels, > 3–5 hours after onset of obstruction, small bowel positioned in centre of abdomen, little or no gas or stool in colon with completes mechanical obstruction after 12–24 hours.

Stretch sign (erectile volvulae connivertes) completely encircle bowel lumen. Step ladder appearance in low obstruction. String of beads indicates peristaltic hyperactivity to overcome mechanical obstruction.

CT scan is accurate up to 78%, which may show small bowel dilution > 2.5 cm.

Small bowel feces (gas bubbles) mixed with particulate matter proximal to obstruction.

Discrepant caliber at transition zone from dilated to non-dilated bowel.

104. a. True   b. True   c. True   d. False   e. True

Focal nodularhyperplasia most patients are asymptomatic and the tumour is discovered incidentally. The tumour is benign and no treatment is indicated.

Maybe multiple in 7%.

Dramatic homogeneous enhancement during arterial phase of enhanced CT.

Central low density scar (one third of the cases).

Cold defect on technechtium-99 sulfur colloid-labeled liver scan (50%).

105. a. True   b. True   c. True   d. False   e. False

Tear is longitudinal and involves the mucosa and submucosa due to raised pressure secondary to vomiting.

106. a. True   b. True   c. True   d. True   e. False

107. a. True   b. True   c. False   d. False   e. False

Candida Esophagitis (Moniliasis)
- Most common cause if infectious esophagitis.
- Usually occurs as an opportunitistic infection in those with depressed immunity, diabetes mellitus, steroids, chemotherapy, and radiotherapy.
- Diseases which cause delayed esophageal emptying scleroderma, strictures, achalasia, and S/P fundoplication.
- Rarely may occur in otherwise healthy individuals.
- Produces whitish slightly raised plaques.
- Symptoms are dysphagia, odynophagia, intense substernal pain, associated with oral thrush (orpharyngeal moniliasis) in 20–80% and predilection for 1/2 of oesophagus.
- Imaging findings double-contrast esophagram may show discrete plaque-like lesions, larger plaques may coalesce to produce 'cobblestone' appearance, further coalescence produces 'shaggy' contour (from coalescent plaques, pseudomembranes, rosions, ulcerations, intramural haemorrhage) in fulminant candidiasis. More fulminant form is more often associated with AIDS.
- Diagnosis
  • Endoscopy most sensitive method of making diagnoasis for mild cases, double-contrasr esophagography should pick up 90% of cases.

108. a. False   b. True   c. True   d. True   e. True

Typical achalasia is characterised by traid of elevated resting lower esophageal sphincter pressure, incomplete relaxation of the sphincter and absence of primary peristalsis in most or all of eosophageal body. The eosuphagus may not be dilated in early achalasia and in a subtype of achalasia called vigorous achalasia.

109. a. False   b. False   c. True   d. False   e. True

110. a. True   b. False   c. True   d. True   e. True

Cushing's disease describes the signs and symptoms associated with prolonged exposure to in appropriately high levels of hormone cortisol.

Mnemonic (CUSHING)
C – central obesity, clavical fat collagen fibre weakness.
U – urinary free cortisol and glucose increase.
S – striae suppressed immunity.
H – hypercortisolism, hypertension, hyperglycemia, hypercholesterolemia, hirtuism, hypernatremia, hypokalemia.
I – iatrogenic (increased administration of corticosteroids).
N- non iatrogenic (neoplasms).
G – glucose intolerance, growth retardation.
- Radiological investigations including chest x-ray, CT scanning of the adrenal gland and MRI for pituitary gland are performed to detect the presence of any adrenal or pituitary or incidentalomas, etc.

111. a. True   b. False   c. True   d. True   e. False

Faster heart rate also causes urinary retention, urticarial, constipation, lowered blood pressure, dry mouth, itching, and others.

112. a. False   b. False   c. True   d. True   e. False

Litter hernia contain Meckel's diverticulum also called persistent omophalomesentric duct hernia. Ritcher's hernia is entrapment of ischemia of antimesentric border of bowel. Spingelian hernia occurs through semi-circular line which is lateral to rectus abdominous muscle. Femoral hernia is more common in female but inguinal hernia is still the most common hernia in female. Anterior peritoneal hernia is through a defect in urogenital membrane and the posterior hernia occurs through a defect in levator ani.

113. a. True   b. False   c. True   d. True   e. True

114. a. False   b. True   c. False   d. True   e. True

Radiological features are no dilatation of the small bowel. Moderately thickened wall of small bowel but not rigid folds nodules are present, hypersecretion, fragmentation, segmentation, normal transit time, hepatosplenomegaly.

115. a. True   b. True   c. False   d. False   e. False

Esophageal Web
Ringlike constriction of upper oesophagus covered on superior and inferior surfaces by squamous epithelium.

Three types have been described:
A non-specific or idiopathic web (most common).

Webs associated with Plummer-Vinson Syndrome

Webs associated with epidermolysis bullosa dystrophica or graft-versus-host disease

Usually found in middle-aged females.

Plummer-Vinson syndrome = Patterson-Kelly syndrome

Iron deficiency anaemia, stomatitis, glossitis, dysphagia, spoon-shaped nails, esophageal webs, and some question as to whether such a syndrome exists.

Cervical oesophagus anteriorly at level of the cricopharyngeous (C5–C6).

Thin, transverse filling defects.

Perpendicular to anterior esophageal wall.

Usually less than 3 mm in thickness.

116. a. True   b. True   c. True   d. True   e. False

117. a. False   b. False   c. True   d. False   e. True

118. a. True   b. True   c. True   d. False   e. False

119. a. True   b. True   c. False   d. True   e. True

120. a. True   b. True   c. False   d. True   e. True

Litter hernia containing meckel diverticulum richter hernia containing on wall of a bowel loop, spigelian hernia also known as lateral ventral hernia. Along the spigelion line between the rectus abdominis muscle and the semillunar line. Foramen of winslow (epiploic foramen)is the passage of communication between the greater and lesser sac. epigastric hernia occur ventrally thriong a defect in linea alba superior the umbilicus known also as a fatty hernia of linea alba commonly in obese or pregnancy.

121. a. True   b. True   c. False   d. False   e. True

Overdistension of the appendix with mucous secondary to luminal obstruction by fecolith, or foreign body endometriosis, or carcinoi. Peripheral rim-like calcification maybe seen even on plain abdominal x-ray or CT scan. May be asymptomic, when rupture may produce pseudomyxoma peritonei.

122. a. False   b. True   c. False   d. False   e. False

Cathartic colon prolong use of laxative results in neuromuscular incoordination from chronically increased muscle activity usually requires more than 10 years of laxative use, e.g., castor oil, podophyllum. Usually involves colon mucosa with smooth flattered surface absent haustration no skip lesion or preudopolyps.

123. a. True   b. True   c. True   d. True   e. False

124. a. True   b. False c. True   d. True   e. True

125. a. True   b. False c. True   d. True   e. False

126. a. True   b. False c. True   d. True   e. True

On CT scan strand-like infiltration of the bowel mesentery producing a haziness seen also in lymphpoma, pancreatitis, tubercolisis.

127. a. True   b. True   c. False   d. True   e. True

128. a. True   b. False   c. True   d. False   e. False

129. a. True   b. True   c. True   d. True   e. False

Also seen in Crohn's disease, celiac disease, cystic fibrosis, eosinophilic gastritis, gastritis menetries disease, carcinoid syndrome, Whipple's disease, mastocytosis, post surgery or infectious or drugs (neomycin), etc.

130. a. True   b. True   c. True   d. False   e. False

It can also occur in the caecum, sigmoid colon. Very soft mass can be impalpable even at laparotomy.

131. a. False   b. True   c. False   d. True   e. True

Double bubble sign is dilated stomach and proximal duodenum. Also seen in superior mesenteric artery syndrome.

132. a. True   b. True   c. False   d. True   e. True

133. a. True   b. True   c. True   d. False   e. True

134. a. False   b. False   c. False   d. False   e. True

Jackstone calculus is a urinary bladder stone with jagged irregular margins indicating formation in a trabeculated bladder.

Mercedes-Benz sign represent tri-radiate appearance of air in gallstone can be seen on plain films.

Popcorn calcification represents flocculent, amorphous calcification in solid masses frequently indicating smooth muscle calcification.

Rice grain calcifications represents elongated oval-shaped, soft tissue calcifications the size of rice grains seen in cysticercosis.

135. a. True   b. True   c. True   d. False   e. True

Other risks factors are gallstone female gender, increasing age, rapid weight loss, hyperlipidemia, and biliary illness.

136. a. True   b. True   c. True   d. False   e. False

137. a. True   b. True   c. True   d. True   e. False

138. a. True   b. False   c. True   d. True   e. True

139. a. True   b. True   c. False   d. True   e. True

Lye stricture, esophageal stricture formation due to ingestion of caustic or corrosive substances.

140. a. False   b. False   c. True   d. True   e. True

141. a. True   b. False   c. True   d. True   e. True

Colon cut off sign the pattern of bowel gas in which there is air in a slightly dilated transverse colon up to, but not beyond the splenic flexure. This sign is seen in CT scan as well as conventional radiography.

142. a. True   b. True   c. False   d. True   e. True

143. a. True   b. True   c. True   d. False   e. True

144. a. True   b. False   c. True   d. False   e. False

Toxic Mega Colon

Potentially lethal dilation of all or part of the colon associated with colitis. Toxic colitis is a clinical diagnosis it may be associated with mega colon. Dilatation of the colon can occur without toxicity. Toxicity of the colon can occur without dilatation of the colon.

Toxic mega colon is due to ulcerative colitis. Ischemic pseudomembranous colitis or inflammatory colitis.

Conventional radiography is usually diagnostic.

Barium enema should not be performed.

145. a. True   b. True   c. True   d. False   e. False

146. a. False   b. True   c. True   d. False   e. True

147. a. True   b. True   c. False   d. True   e. True

148. a. True   b. True   c. True   d. True   e. False

149. a. True   b. False   c. True   d. True   e. False

150. a. True   b. True   c. False   d. True   e. True

151. a. False b. True   c. True   d. True   e. False

152. a. True   b. True   c. False   d. True   e. True

153. a. True   b. False c. False   d. True   e. True

154. a. True   b. False c. True   d. True   e. True

155. a. True   b. False c. False   d. False e. False

Desmoid Tumour
Greek word 'desmos', which means tendon-like, is benign, noninflammatory fibroblastic tumour with tendency to local invasion and recurrence but without metastasis. Most frequently encountered between 20 and 40 years. More in woman. Most common arise from the rectus abdominus muscles. Some cases associated with oestrogen therapy. Also associated with familial adenomatous polyposis.

On ultrasound, typically appear as homogeneously anechoic or hypoechoic masses.

On CT images most are relatively homogeneously or focally hyperattenuating. When compared with the soft tissue on the non contrast scan and demonstrate some enhancement following IV contrast.

On MRI, low signal intensity on T1 and on T2 as well.

156. a. True   b. True   c. True   d. False e. True

157. a. True   b. True   c. False   d. True   e. True

Pneumatosis cystoides intestinalis is presence of gas in the bowel wall can be seen in chronic obstructive pulmonary disease, e.g., ruptured blebs allows air to dissect down through retroperitoneum tthrough mesentery to serosa or submucosa.

Also seen in obstruction of the GIT, e.g., pyloric stenosis, Hirchsprung's disease or carcinoma of the bowel with obstruction. some inflammatory disease includingnecrotinizing enterocolitis, ingestion of caustic materials, and mesenteric ischemia.

Secondary form occurs mostly in small bowel may mimic polyps when they protrude into lumen, however usually linear and streak-like rather cystic, the lucency of air are parallels bowel wall.

158. a. True   b. True   c. False   d. True   e. True

159. a. True   b. True   c. False   d. True   e. True

Mesenteric vein thrombosis also seen in Crohn's, ulcerative colitis, birth control pills, trauma, etc.

160. a. True   b. True   c. True   d. True   e. False

Also seen in superior and inferior vena cava thrombosis.

161. a. True   b. True   c. True   d. False   e. True

Others intestinal lymphagectasia, nonspecific granuloma. Ligation or damage to thoracic duct. The tropical sprue is a cause of protein-losing enteropathy but not due to lymphatic.

162. a. True   b. True   c. False   d. False   e. True

163. a. False   b. False   c. True   d. True   e. False

164. a. False   b. False   c. False   d. True   e. True

165. a. True   b. True   c. True   d. False   e. True

166. a. True   b. False   c. True   d. True   e. True

167. a. False   b. False   c. False   d. True   e. True

Quadrate lobe is representing the medial segment of the left lobe of the liver (segment IV). The caudate lobe is (segment one). The Reidel's lobe is accessory hepatic lobe are normal variants related to the right extend caudal.

168. a. True   b. True   c. False   d. True   e. True

Omental cake refer to infiltration of the omental fat by material of soft tissue density. May also be seen in lymphadenoma and malignant ascities.

169. a. True   b. True   c. True   d. True   e. False

170. a. False   b. True   c. False   d. True   e. False

It is transient ridge diagnosed by barium swallow.

171. a. True   b. True   c. True   d. False   e. True

172. a. True   b. True   c. True   d. True   e. False

173. a. True   b. True   c. True   d. True   e. False

174. a. True   b. True   c. False   d. True   e. False

175. a. False   b. True   c. True   d. True   e. True

Ectopic pancreas, aberrant or hetrotopic parirentic tissue, which is oftenly referred as pancreatic rest can be found anywhere along the foregut and proximal midgut. About 75% of all pancreatic rests are located in the stomach, duodenum, or jejunum.

176. a. True   b. True   c. True   d. True   e. False

177. a. True   b. False   c. False   d. False   e. False

178. a. False   b. True   c. True   d. False   e. True

179. a. True   b. True   c. False   d. True   e. False

180. a. True   b. True   c. True   d. True   e. False

181. a. True   b. True   c. True   d. False   e. False

182. a. False   b. True   c. False   d. True   e. False

183. a. False   b. True   c. True   d. True   e. True

184. a. False   b. True   c. True   d. False   e. False

Intramural pseudodiverticulosis of the oesophagus is a rare condition, represents barium filling the excretory ducts of the mucus glands of the oesophagus. These mucus glands are normal anatomic structures of the oesophagus but typically are not visible on radiologic studies.

Sometimes these ducts become dilated, allowing barium to track into the ducts and glands. Candida organism is found as a secondary infection of the glands.

Dysphagia lusoria is seen in Aberrent right subclavian artery when the long length oblique impression of the oesophagus just below the aortic knuckle by the artery.

185. a. True   b. True   c. False   d. True   e. True

186. a. True   b. False   c. False   d. False   e. False

A true diverticulum that includes all three coats of the small intestine, 40–90 cm proximal to the ileocecal valve in location. May contains heterotropic tissue (gastric mucosa) in about 50%.

Occurs in about 2% of general population.

187. a. True   b. True   c. True   d. True   e. False

188. a. True   b. True   c. False   d. True   e. True

189. a. True   b. True   c. False   d. False   e. True

190. a. True   b. True   c. True   d. False   e. True

191. a. False   b. False   c. True   d. True   e. True

192. a. True   b. True   c. False   d. True   e. False

193. a. True   b. True   c. False   d. False   e. False

194. a. True   b. True   c. False   d. False   e. False.

195. a. True   b. True   c. True   d. False   e. False

Fibrosis of the mediastinum or bulky adenopathy can produce downhill varices so as thrombosis of the superior vena cava.

196. a. False   b. False   c. False   d. True   e. False

Angiodysplasia is a disease of the colon commonly affected the right colon than the left of unknown aetiology, presented with painless gastro intestinal tract bleeding. Diagnosed best by angiogram. Commonly affects elderly male patient.

197. a. False   b. True   c. True   d. True   e. True

Menetries disease is a benign lesion of the stomach. Thickened gastric folds marked glandular hypertrophy of the stomach. Is differs from eosinophilic gastritis not respond to steroid.

1. Homonymous hemianopia may be seen in:
   a) Craniopharyngioma.
   b) Optic tract lesion.
   c) Fibrous dysplasia of the skull base.
   d) Aneurysm of anterior communication artery.
   e) Demyelination.
2. In lacunar skull:
   a) Affected the outer table of the skull vault commonly.
   b) The occipital bone is commonly affected.
   c) Associated with spina bifida oculta.
   d) Present at birth.
   e) Chiari II malformation is recognized association.
3. Sclerosis of the base of the skull may occur with:
   a) Paget's disease.
   b) Osteopetrosis.
   c) Neurofibromatosis.
   d) Tuberculosis.
   e) Fibrous dysplasia.

4. The following are features of juvenile angiofibroma:
   a) Simulates adenoid enlargement on lateral plain view.
   b) Causes erosion of the floor of sphenoid sinus.
   c) More common in females.
   d) Characteristics angiographic appearance.
   e) Rarely bleeds.

5. Rubella embryopathy may show:
   a) Deafness.
   b) Cataract.
   c) Spina bifida.
   d) Excretion of living virus for several months after birth.
   e) Periosteal reactions.

6. In cranial nerve palsy:
   a) Chronic suppurative otitis media.
   b) Acoustic neuroma.
   c) Fractured petrous bone.
   d) Parotid carcinoma.
   e) Aneurysm post communicating artery.

7. Ranulas the following are true:
   a) Abscess collection in the parotid region.
   b) Associated with lymphoma.
   c) Associated with histocytosis.
   d) Associated with mandibular osteomyelitis.
   e) Plunging ranula usually extended below the level of the myelohyoid.

8. The following give rise to a paraspinal mass:
   a) Sickle cell anaemia.
   b) Portal hypertension.
   c) Sarcoid.
   d) Hypertrophic oesteoarthropathy.
   e) Myeloma.

9. Spina bifida oculta may be seen in:
   a) Obese mother during pregnancy.
   b) Diabetic mother during pregnancy.
   c) Carbamazepine medication mother during pregnancy.
   d) Diastematomyelia.
   e) Myelosclerosis.

10. Specific complications of Truncal Vagotomy:
    a) Dysphagia.
    b) Diarrhoea.
    c) Postural hypotension.

d) Gastric stasis.
e) Cardiac arrhythmias.

11. The following are true in neuroblastoma:
    a) Hyperglycemia.
    b) Acute cerebral encephalopathy may occur.
    c) Bone metastasis is rare.
    d) Diarrhoea about 9%.
    e) Sparing the pelvis.

12. In Tullio's phenomenon are true:
    a) Digital volume tomography is the examination of choice.
    b) Scleroderma is usually associated condition.
    c) Female between 10 and 20 years is usual age.
    d) Conductive hearing loss.
    e) Oscillopsia.

13. The following are in favour of optic sheath meningioma rather than optic glioma:
    a) Bilateral.
    b) Middle-aged women.
    c) Orbital hyperostosis.
    d) Widened optic canal.
    e) Calcification on CT scan.

14. In subarachnoid haemorrhage (SAH):
    a) Commonly in children.
    b) Bloody spinal fluid.
    c) Enhanced CT scan is the study of choice.
    d) Confusion.
    e) Communicating hydrocephalus seen in acute cases.

15. In subdural haematoma:
    a) Spread all over the cerebral surface in the infants.
    b) In children become localised around and below temporal lobe.
    c) In adult there is clear history of trauma usually.
    d) On CT scan classically cresentic shape.
    e) In acute cases papillary abnormalities seen in less than 10% of the cases.

16. Tuberculous meningitis:
    a) May be accompanied by miliary TB.
    b) May be associated with a negative tuberculin test.
    c) Is an indication for intrathecal isoniazid.
    d) Should be treated routinely with corticosteroids as well as chemotherapy.
    e) Enhanced meningies by CT scan.

17. Which of the following are features of Bechet's syndrome:
    a) Thrombophlebitis.
    b) Light sensitivity.
    c) Premature senility.
    d) Xerostomia.
    e) Uvetis.

18. In patients with cerebral angiomas:
    a) May show increased skull markings.
    b) Early venous filling.
    c) Intracranial calcification.
    d) Erosion of the dorsum sella.
    e) Cerebral atrophy.

19. Frontal bossing seen in:
    a) Achondroplasia.
    b) Anaemia.
    c) Mucopolysaccharidosis.
    d) Mongolism.
    e) Hydroencephaly.

20. In epidermoids:
    a) Have a well-defined margin.
    b) Occur only in the skull.
    c) May occur in the orbital roof.
    d) May show radiating spicules.
    e) Have atypical vascular pattern.

21. In meningioma:
    a) May be found anywhere throughout the nervous sytem.
    b) Usually calcified tumour.
    c) Highly enhanced by CT scan.

d) Always benign.
e) Common in males of less 30 years of age.

22. In medulloblastoma:
    a) Medulloblastoma most common paediatric posterior fossa tumour.
    b) Medulloblastoma seeds down the spine.
    c) Associated with Gardner syndrome.
    d) Calcification occurs in 80%.
    e) It shows hypointense to grey matter on T1.

23. Single radiolucent bone defect on plain skull x-ray seen in:
    a) Leptomeningeal cyst.
    b) Burr hole.
    c) Cholesteatoma.
    d) Brown tumour.
    e) Crouzon's disease.

24. J-shape sella on lateral skull x-ray seen in:
    a) Cretinism.
    b) Gargolism.
    c) Optic chiasma glioma.
    d) Always abnormal.
    e) Usually associated with high intracranial pressure.

25. There is recognised association between neurofibromatosis and:
    a) Phaechromocytoma.
    b) Coarctation of the abdominal aorta.
    c) Pseudo-arthrosis of the tibia.
    d) Wide interpedicular distance in the lumbar spine.
    e) Extramedullary haemopoiesis.

26. Thickening of the skull vault is found in:
    a) Tuberculosis.
    b) Myotonia dystrophica.
    c) Acromegaly.
    d) Hypothyroidism.
    e) Severe chronic anaemia.

27. Thinning of the skull vault found in:
    a) Craniolacunia.
    b) Progeria.
    c) Thalassemia.
    d) Pyle's disease.
    e) Neurofibromatosis.

28. There is an increase in lumbar interpedicular distance in:
    a) Diastematomyelia.
    b) Spina bifida without meningocoele.
    c) Ependymoma.
    d) Achondroplasia.
    e) Osteitis condensans ilii.

29. Calcification in the region of the pituitary fossa may be on plain radiograph seen in:
    a) An optic nerve glioma.
    b) Craniopharyngioma.
    c) Chromophobe adenoma.
    d) Carotid siphon.
    e) Petro clinoid ligament.

30. Rarefaction of the dorsum sella is present in:
    a) Mucopolysaccharidosis.
    b) Cystic fibrosis.
    c) Senility.
    d) Benign raised intracranial pressure.
    e) Malignant hypertension.

31. Unilateral exophthalmus can be due to:
    a) Subdural haemorrhage.
    b) Osteoma is orbito ethmoidal region.
    c) Mucocoele of ethmoid.
    d) Cavernous sinus thrombosis.
    e) Orbital varices.

32. Wormain bones occur in:
    a) Hyperphosphastasia.
    b) Trauma.
    c) Rickets.

d) Osteogenesis imperfecta.
e) Progeria.

33. Obstructive hydrocephalus seen in:
    a) Colloid cyst.
    b) Dandy-Walker cyst.
    c) Archnoid cyst.
    d) Choroid plexus papilloma.
    e) Distematomyelia.

34. In inverted papilloma:
    a) Ostiomeatal unit obstruction is featured.
    b) CECT scan shows lobulated tumour surface.
    c) Associated with juvenile angiofibroma.
    d) T1C+MR shows an enhancing mass in the middle meatus with extension into the maxillary and/or the ethmoid sinus.
    e) The cerebriform mixed enhancement within the sinus cavity is a feature on CECT scan.

35. In subdural hematoma:
    a) In infants occupies the whole subdural space.
    b) Without midline shift indicates ipsilateral cerebral atrophy.
    c) In adults is always associated with a history of trauma.
    d) Tends to collect below the temporal lobe.
    e) MRI is more informative than CT scan.

36. Basal ganglia calcification seen in:
    a) Parkinsonism.
    b) Fahr's syndrome.
    c) Pseudo hypoparathyroidism.
    d) Multipara.
    e) Arnoid-Chiari malformation.

37. In macrocephaly occurs in:
    a) Subdural haematoma.
    b) Achondroplasia.
    c) Dandy-Walker syndrome.
    d) Subarachnoid cyst.
    e) Aqueduct stenosis.

38. In diplopia:
    a) Associated with Grave's disease.
    b) Myasthenia.
    c) Multiple sclerosis.
    d) Guillian-Barre syndrome.
    e) Pansinusitis.

39. Basilar impression seen in:
    a) Histocytosis X.
    b) Arnold-Chiari malformation.
    c) Hypervitaminosis D.
    d) Fluorosis.
    e) Rheumatoid arthritis.

40. Localised hyperostosis of the calvarium seen in:
    a) Haemangioma.
    b) Meningioma.
    c) Osteoma.
    d) Acoustic neuroma.
    e) Plexiform neurofibroma.

41. The lamina dura around the teeth is lost in:
    a) Paget's disease.
    b) Fibrous dysplasia.
    c) Senile osteoporosis.
    d) Hypopituitarism.
    e) Scurvy.

42. A patient with progressive unilateral involvement of cranial nerves 3, 4, 5, 6, 9, 10 and sphenoid destruction may have:
    a) Juvenile angiofibroma.
    b) Chordoma of clivus.
    c) Nasopharyngeal carcinoma.
    d) Craniopharygioma.
    e) Glomus jugular tumour.

43. Optic canal enlargement seen in:
    a) Chiasmatic archnoiditis.
    b) Lacrimal gland carcinoma.
    c) Hurler syndrome.

d) Meningioma of optic nerve sheath.
e) Retinoblastoma.

44. The following are features of carcinoma of larynx:
    a) Subglottic is a common site.
    b) Glottic carcinoma is detected early due to hoarseness.
    c) Glottic tumours have best prognosis.
    d) Cervical gland involvement occurs earlier in supraglottic than in subglottic.
    e) Smoking and alcohol abuse are risk factors.

45. In MRI, expansion of the cord shadow may be due to:
    a) Tabes dorsalis.
    b) Disc protrusion.
    c) Ependymoma.
    d) Disseminated sclerosis.
    e) Syringomyelia.

46. In spontaneous intracranial hypotention (SIH).
    a) Peak prevalence is in the third and fourth decades.
    b) The classic presentation is orthostatic headache.
    c) May presented with encephalopathy.
    d) Normal CT scan in the majority of the cases.
    e) MRI finding, there is diffuse brain swelling, sagging brain stem.

47. Multiple intracranial calcifications are found in:
    a) Myelosclerosis.
    b) Neurofibromatosis.
    c) Histoplasmosis.
    d) Toxoplasmosis.
    e) Tuberculosis.

48. Cerebrellopontine angle mass seen in:
    a) Neuroma V nerve.
    b) Neuroma IIV nerve.
    c) TB meningitis.
    d) Chordoma.
    e) Acoustic neuroma.

49. Atlanto-axial dislocation in children occurs in:
    a) Still's disease.
    b) Down syndrome.
    c) Morquio's disease.
    d) Lupus erythematosus.
    e) Retropharyngeal abscess.

50. In empty sella syndrome:
    a) Incidence 10% of population.
    b) Common in male.
    c) Increase the risk of CSF Rhinorrhea.
    d) Endocranial anomality is common.
    e) May be secondary to disruption of the diaphragma sellae surgically.

51. Intracranial pneumocephalus seen in:
    a) Mucocele.
    b) Mastoiditis.
    c) Osteoma of the frontal sinuses.
    d) Brain stem glioma.
    e) Pleomorphic xanthoastrocytoma.

52. The coronal clefts seen in neonatal vertebra:
    a) Represent the site of nutrient vessels.
    b) Are commonest in the upper dorsal region.
    c) May be used to delineate the extent of a spina bifida.
    d) May be seen pre-natally.
    e) Represent venous sinusoid.

53. Posterior mediastinal lesion may be due to:
    a) Bochdalek hernia.
    b) Neuroenteric cyst.
    c) Pheochromocytoma.
    d) Thymoma.
    e) Thoracic kidney.

54. In hypervitaminosis D:
    a) Widening of the provisional zone of calcification.
    b) Dense Calvarium.
    c) Nephrocalcinosis.

d) Looser's zone is likely present.
   e) Premature calcification of fax cerebri.

55. Sclerosis of the skull in child is associated:
    a) Osteopathia striata.
    b) Turner's syndrome.
    c) Engelmann's disease.
    d) Fibrous dysplasia.
    e) Cleidocranial dysostosis.

56. In angiofibroma of the nasopharynx:
    a) Commonly in female.
    b) May erode the sphenoid sinus.
    c) Can be mistaken for adenoids.
    d) Usually associated with bone tumour.
    e) Angiography is superb over the CT scan.

57. Which of the following are recognised associations:
    a) Marfan's syndrome and aortic dissection.
    b) Klippel-Feil syndrome and inner ear anomalies.
    c) Reiter's syndrome and aortic valve incompetence.
    d) Hyper telorism and Down syndrome.
    e) Oesophageal stenosis and epidermolysis bullosa.

58. Limbus vertebra are true:
    a) Commonly affected a single vertebra.
    b) Not associated with a schmoral's node.
    c) Seen mostly in the mid-lumber spine.
    d) Posterior limbus vertebra may causes nerve compression.
    e) Can be seen in the cervical spine.

59. Extradural abscess over the petrous bone may be associated with:
    a) Purulent cerebrospinal fluid.
    b) Upward shift of pineal body.
    c) Middle ear infection.
    d) 5th nerve involvement.
    e) 3rd nerve involvement.

60. Underdeveloped sinuses commonly occur in:
    a) Treatcher Collins syndrome.
    b) Thalassemia.

c) Marfan's syndrome.
   d) Osteopetrosis.
   e) Down syndrome.

61. Separation or infiltration of skull sutures in an infant or child seen in:
    a) Neuroblastoma metastasis.
    b) Wilm's tumour metastasis.
    c) Hygroma.
    d) Lead poisoning.
    e) Hypervitaminosis D.

62. Thickening of the skull vault is commonly seen in:
    a) Basal cell nevus syndrome.
    b) Congenital indifference to pain (Asymbolia).
    c) Treated hydrocephalus.
    d) Myotonic dystrophy.
    e) Mucopolysaccharidosis I-H (Huler's).

63. In Klippel-Feil syndrome:
    a) There may be upper dorsal rib anomalies.
    b) May be associated with Sprengel's deformity.
    c) There may be abnormality of cervical spinal cord.
    d) Respiratory distress may occur.
    e) Renal agenesis may be associated.

64. There is well-recognised association between neurofibromatosis:
    a) J-shaped sella.
    b) Optic glioma.
    c) Carotid A. Stenosis.
    d) Cranial manifestation in the neonatal period.
    e) Precociuos puberty.

65. The following statements are true:
    a) The aerated maxillary antra are usually visible by 3 m of age.
    b) The ethmoid air cells are usually aerated by 3 m.
    c) The Spheroid sinuses are usually aerated by 5 years.
    d) A pan-sinusitis may present with exopthalmus.
    e) The frontal sinuses are usually aerated by 2 years.

66. The following statements are true:
    a) Hypoplasia of the mandible is a feature of mandibular facial dysostosis.
    b) There is an association between mandibular hypoplasia and cor pulmonale in infants.
    c) The prognosis of the patient with mandibular hypoplasia is poor.
    d) The position of the patient with mandibular hypoplasia is important.
    e) Respiratory distress does not occur with macroglossia.

67. Which of the following statements is true:
    a) Lung cavitation is more common in secondary than in primary neoplasms.
    b) Myeloma affects the mandible more often than secondary neoplasm.
    c) Pedicle destruction is more often due to myeloma than secondary neoplasm.
    d) Large extra-pleural masses are found in myeloma.
    e) Myelomatosis can give rise to osteoblastic lesion.

68. The following are features of cysticerocis:
    a) Is caused by eating infected pork.
    b) Cysts in liver and spleen are transonic on ultrasonic examination.
    c) A complement fixation test in diagnostic.
    d) Tiny calcifications may occur in the brain.
    e) The lungs are not usually involved without liver involvement.

69. The following masses occur in the posterior mediastinum:
    a) Lipoma.
    b) Cystic hygroma.
    c) Ganglioneuroma.
    d) Dermoid.
    e) Bronchogenic cyst.

70. Atlanto-axial subluxation seen in adults:
    a) Retropharyngeal abscess in children.
    b) Mongolism.
    c) Ankylosing spondylitis.
    d) Diastrophic dwarfism.
    e) Cretinism.

71. Large orbit seen in:
    a) Pseudotumour.
    b) Neurofibromatosis.
    c) Varix of orbital vein.
    d) Radiation therapy.
    e) Enucleation.

72. Unilateral exophthalmos seen in:
    a) Histocytosis.
    b) Paget's disease.
    c) Mucocele.
    d) Sjogren's syndrome.
    e) Thalassemia.

73. In early subacute cerebral hematoma the following are true:
    a) The time period is up to 14 days.
    b) High density lesion within the 1st week on unenhanced CT scan.
    c) Very hyperintense on T1W1.
    d) Very hyperintense on T2W1.
    e) Central rim is isotense on T2.

74. Generalised convulsions following injection of contrast should be treated by:
    a) Pentothal.
    b) Calcium gluconate.
    c) Adrenaline.
    d) Coramine.
    e) Ventilation.

75. The following are true in laryngeal papillomas:
    a) Associated with genital warts.
    b) Associated with tracheal papilloma in more than 25%.
    c) Lateral view of the neck may show a calcified mass at prevertebral space within the larynges region.
    d) Diagnosis is made using flexible fibrotic laryngoscopy.
    e) Commonly in female with painful hoarseness.

76. The following are true in rhabdomyosarcoma:
    a) Can arise anywhere in the body.
    b) Locally malignant.

c) Commonly presented at 1ˢᵗ decade of life.
d) Head and neck are common location.
e) Associated with Turner's syndrome.

77. In mucocele of frontal sinus:
    a) Headaches.
    b) Diplopia.
    c) Increased translucency on plain x-ray.
    d) Associated with osteoma.
    e) Hypertelorism.

78. Microcephaly seen in:
    a) Phenylketonuria.
    b) Hemocystinuria.
    c) Aminoaciduria.
    d) Ferrocalcinosis.
    e) Dandy-Walker syndrome.

79. Widened interpedicular distance in the lumbar region seen in:
    a) Neurofibromatosis.
    b) Achondroplasia.
    c) Mucopolysacharidosis.
    d) Syringomyelia.
    e) Diastematomyelia.

80. Brucellosis is associates with:
    a) Neutrophic leukocytosis.
    b) Hypertrophic osteoarthropathy.
    c) Meningitis.
    d) Lobar consolidation.
    e) Chronic osteomyelitis.

81. Intraorbital calcifications found in:
    a) Phleboliths.
    b) Orbital meningioma.
    c) Thyroid-eye disease.
    d) Lacrimal gland malignancy.
    e) Retinoblastoma.

82. In limierre syndrome:
    a) Intracranial septic emboli are likely present.
    b) Pain in the mandible on the affected side.
    c) Contrasts enhance CT scan is the imaging study of choice.
    d) Associated with rheumatoid arthritis.
    e) Atlanto-axial dislocation may be present.

83. The following are true in hygroma:
    a) It is premalignant.
    b) In the neck, the posterior cervical space is frequent location.
    c) The mediastinum is a possible site.
    d) Sparing the retroperitoneal organs.
    e) Can involve the scrotum.

84. The following are true in vein of Galen malformation:
    a) Generalised dilatation of head and neck vessels.
    b) Oligemic lungs.
    c) Hydrocephalus.
    d) Steal phenomenon on echocardiography.
    e) Associated with pneumomediastinum.

85. Bone tumours favouring vertebral bodies than posterior elements are:
    a) Ewing sarcoma.
    b) Metastasis from the breast.
    c) Chondrosarcoma.
    d) Osteoid osteoma.
    e) Haemangioma.

86. The following are true in eosinophilic granuloma:
    a) May be presented with otitis media.
    b) Diabetes insipidus.
    c) Honeycomb lungs.
    d) Vertebra planna.
    e) The disease is sparing the skull vault.

87. Moya-moya is true:
    a) Familial in Japan.
    b) Common in black children with sickle cell anaemia.
    c) In childhood TIAs and strokes are common.
    d) Associated with tubersclerosis.
    e) Common in transplacental infection.

88. In fibromuscular dysplasia (hyperplasia):
    a) Commonly young male between 3 and 25 years.
    b) Hypertension is common.
    c) Can find in any location including carotid arteries.
    d) Diagnosed confidently by CT angiogram and/or MRI.
    e) Can cause intracranial aneurysm.

89. In dislocations of the mandible:
    a) Common in Marfan's syndrome.
    b) Can occur during seizure.
    c) Prognathic appearance to jaw indicates both sides are dislocated.
    d) CT scan is good diagnostic modality.
    e) Associated with Atlanto-axial dislocation in the majority of the cases in traumatic cases.

90. In haemangioma of the spine are true:
    a) Potentially malignant.
    b) Vertebral body is increase in size.
    c) Thickened vertebral trabeculae can be seen on plain radiograph of the spine.
    d) Increased signal intensity on both T1 and T2.
    e) Indistinguishable from multiple myeloma by nuclear medicine.

91. The following are true in retropharengeal abscess:
    a) May be associated with middle ear infection.
    b) Cervical lyphadenopathy is rare.
    c) Is a disease of teen age group.
    d) Can cause jugular vein thrombosis.
    e) Surgical drainage is contraindication.

92. In epiglottitis the following are true:
    a) Mean age 3–5 years.
    b) Abrupt onset of stridor often associated with dysphagia.
    c) Emergency tracheal intubation to prevent airway obstruction and respiratory failure.
    d) Most common etiologic agent is group A streptococcus.
    e) It may be due to bee stings.

93. The following are true in enlarged tonsils:
    a) Lymphoma.
    b) Enlarged tonsils may be seen when dynamic imaging studies are performed to evaluate for obstructive sleep apnea.
    c) Hepatitis (A) viruses.
    d) During infancy.
    e) Large adenoid tonsils can completely obstruct the nasopharynx.

94. Floating teeth occur in:
    a) Gout.
    b) Papillon-LeFever syndrome (Juvenile periodontosis).
    c) Langerhan's cell histiocytosis.
    d) Acromegaly.
    e) Hyperparathyroidism.

95. In craniosynostosis:
    a) Premature fusion of the sagittal suture is commonly affected.
    b) Brain growth is the major factor in keeping sutures open.
    c) Oxycephaly when all skull suture and basilar fused early.
    d) Associated with apert syndrome.
    e) Due to vitamin D deficiency.

96. In paranasal osteoma:
    a) Associated with colonic polyps.
    b) Associated with skin lesions.
    c) Sparing the mandible.
    d) May be associated with Paget's disease.
    e) May be presented with cerebrospinal fluid Rhinorrhea.

97. In sialolithiasis:
    a) Usually involve the parotid gland.
    b) Usually radiolucent.
    c) Associated with hyperparathyroidism.
    d) The location of the stone in the course of Stensen's duct when the submandibular gland involve.
    e) Sialography is contraindicated in acute infection of the gland.

98. Calcification occurs in more than 5% of the following:
    a) Pituitary adenoma.
    b) Craniopharyngioma.
    c) Cerebral metastases.

d) Optic glioma.
e) Astrocytoma.

99. Small or abscent sinuses occur in:
    a) Cretinism
    b) Arteriovenous malformations
    c) Down's syndrome
    d) Acromegaly
    e) Kartagener's syndrome

100. In thyroid opthamopathy:
     a) May be unilateral.
     b) Associated with pretibial edema.
     c) Focal thyroid enlargement on ultrasound is usually present.
     d) CT scan shows enlargement of the extraocular muscles with sparing of the tendons.
     e) Hyperemic thyroid on color Doppler.

101. In retinoblastoma;
     a) Common in neonate.
     b) Benign tumor.
     c) Avascular.
     d) Can be bilateral.
     e) leukocoria.

102. In extramedullary haematopoiesis in thalassemia:
     a) Bilateral paraspinal masses with round, lobulated margins.
     b) Splenomegaly.
     c) Most often asymptomatic.
     d) Renal failure is common.
     e) Spinal cord compression.

103. Alcoholism has a recognised association with:
     a) Obstructive cardiomyopathy.
     b) Widened cerebral sulci on a CT brain scan.
     c) Ischemic necrosis of the femoral head.
     d) Klebsiella pneumoniae.
     e) Hydrocephalus in the fetus.

104. Diabetes insipidus may be associated with:
    a) Craniopharyngioma.
    b) Pheochromocytoma.
    c) Bronchogenic carcinoma.
    d) Frontal lobe glioma.
    e) Sarcoidosis.

105. Abnormalities of the foramen magnum may occur with:
    a) Cleidocranial dysostosis.
    b) Atlanto occipital fusion.
    c) Plagiocephaly.
    d) Achondroplasia.
    e) The Arnold-Chiari malformation.

106. In the Arnold-Chiari malformation:
    a) The fourth ventricle is low.
    b) The changes are well shown by vertebral angiography.
    c) There is widening of the upper cervical spine.
    d) The plain film is normal.
    e) MRI is the best diagnostic modality.

107. In discitis:
    a) Most common pathogen is staphylococcus.
    b) Usually involvement of one disc space.
    c) Early end plate sclerosis indicating non-pyogenic agent.
    d) Paravertebral soft tissue mass on CT scan seen.
    e) Bacteria destroy disk and both contiguous end plate.

108. In Fahr's disease:
    a) Progressive dementia.
    b) Dysartheria.
    c) Unilateral basal ganglia calcification.
    d) Basal ganglia calcification is rare.
    e) Dentate nuclei calcification is rare.

109. Vertebral pneumatocysts seen in:
    a) Osteomyelitis.
    b) Osteonecrosis.
    c) Myelosclerosis.
    d) Iatrogenic trauma.
    e) Necrotic neoplasm.

110. In hypoxic-ischaemic brain injury (global hypoxic – ischemic injury):
    a) Confined to neonates.
    b) Sparring the grey matter structures.
    c) Generalised brain atrophy.
    d) Diffusion-weighted MR imaging is the earliest imaging modality to become positive within the first few hours after a hypoxic ischaemic event.
    e) CT scan is usually negative.

111. In Wernicke-Korsakoff syndrome:
    a) May be seen after gastric surgery.
    b) CT scan is usually normal.
    c) Commonly affect alcoholic patient.
    d) Associated with active pulmonary tuberculosis.
    e) Opthalmoplegia.

112. The following are true in epidermoid cyst in the skull:
    a) Multiple.
    b) Premalignant.
    c) May communicate with sinuses.
    d) Associated with Klippel-Feil syndrome.
    e) May involve the dural sinuses.

113. In choronid plexus xanthogranuloma:
    a) Malignant tumour.
    b) Hydrocephalus.
    c) Meningitis.
    d) Located in the trigones of the lateral ventricles and bilateral in two-third of the cases.
    e) Usually have high signal on diffusion-weighted imaging and show restriction.

114. In SMART syndrome (Stroke-like-Migraine Attacks After Radiation Therapy):
    a) Early complication of cerebral radiation therapy.
    b) Seizures.
    c) Tension headache.
    d) On MRI, cortical thickening in T2 and flair with diffusion restriction.
    e) Skin pigmentation.

115. In hypertensive encephalopathy (Posterior reversible encephalopathy syndrome):
    a) May be presented with visual disturbance.
    b) Affected regions are hypoattenuating on CT scan.
    c) Hypointense in affected regions on T1.
    d) T2 shows hyperintense in affected regions.
    e) Associated with gliomatosis cerebri.

116. Dandy-Walker malformation may shows:
    a) Vermian agenosis.
    b) Posterior fossa cyst.
    c) Abnormal corpus callosum.
    d) Anterior fossa cyst.
    e) Hydrocephalus.

117. In medulloblastoma:
    a) Midline posterior fossa tumour in paediatric population.
    b) About quarter of the tumour will calcify.
    c) Hydrocephalus is common.
    d) Tendency for drop-seed metastasis.
    e) More common than glioma in the posterior fossa.

118. In spina bifida (neural tube defect/spinal dysraphism):
    a) Most common congenital CNS malformation.
    b) Occur only along the lumbar spine.
    c) Dysplasia of the hip joint.
    d) Neurogenic bladder is common.
    e) Spina bifida cystica associate with Chiari II malformation.

119. In apert syndrome:
    a) Hypotelorism.
    b) Congenital cardiac anomalies.
    c) Symphalangism.
    d) Syndactyly.
    e) Brachycephaly.

120. Base of the skull foramen transmits the following:
    a) Foramen ovale transmits the mandibular nerve branch of trigeminal nerve.
    b) Foramen rotundum transmits maxillary nerve branch of trigeminal nerve.

c) Foramen spinosum transmits the middle meningeal artery.
d) Foramen lacerum transmits the internal carotid artery.
e) Vidian canal transmits the jugular vein.

121. The following are true:
    a) Sialectasis occurs in Sjogren's syndrome.
    b) Primary TB of the lung does not cavitate.
    c) Enlarged temporal fossa occurs in herpes encephalitis.
    d) Constrictive pericarditis is associated with protein losing entropathy.
    e) Menetrier's disease is associated with renal calculi.

122. In rhabdomyosarcema:
    a) Rhabdomyosarcema are found essentially anywhere in the body except the middle ear.
    b) In children and adolescent they occur predominantly in the head, neck, and pelvis.
    c) Associated with neurofibromatosis (NF1).
    d) Maternal use of cocaine and/or marijuana.
    e) On MRI T1C+: shows considerable enhancement/T2; hyperintense prominent flow void maybe seen particularly in extremity lesions.

123. Macrocephaly seen in:
    a) Dandy-Walker syndrome.
    b) Neurofibromatosis.
    c) Hyperphosphatasia.
    d) Fanconi syndrome (aminociduria).
    e) Mucopolysaccharidosis.

124. Microcephaly (Microcrania) seen in:
    a) Homocystine uria.
    b) Phenylketonuria.
    c) Dandy-Walker syndrome.
    d) Prenatal irradiation.
    e) Cat-cry syndrome.

125. Prognathism seen in:
    a) Acromegaly.
    b) Basal cell nevus syndrome (Gorlin).
    c) Hyperparathyroidism.

d) Endentulous mandible.
e) Cherubism.

126. Intra orbital calcifications seen in:
    a) Hypervitaminosis D.
    b) Intra orbital meningioma.
    c) Kartagener's syndrome.
    d) Lacrimal gland carcinoma.
    e) Phthisis bulbi.

127. Small orbit seen in:
    a) Craniostenosis of coronal suture.
    b) Anophthalmos.
    c) Pseudotumour of the orbit.
    d) Thyrotoxicosis.
    e) Fibrous dysplasia.

128. Macroglossia (large tongue) seen in:
    a) Infant of diabetic mother.
    b) Lynphangioma.
    c) Acromegaly.
    d) Addison's disease.
    e) Ochronosis.

129. Large orbit seen in:
    a) Varix of orbital vein.
    b) Optic nerve glioma.
    c) Osteopetrosis.
    d) Congenital glaucoma.
    e) Retinoblastoma.

130. Salivary gland enlargement seen in:
    a) Addison's disease.
    b) Sjogren's syndrome.
    c) Mucoviscitosis (fibrocystic disease of pancreas/cystic fibrosis).
    d) Pregnancy.
    e) Diabetes.

131. Reversal sign on brain CT images is also called (white cerebellum sign) seen in:
    a) Hot nose sign.
    b) Pancake brain sign.
    c) Lemon sign.
    d) Hyperdense MCA sign.
    e) Medusa head sign.

132. In ice cream cone sign.
    a) Represents the normal appearance of the malleus and incus on an axial high-resolution CT scan images of the temporal bone.
    b) The ball 'scoop' of the ice cream is formed by the head of the malleus.
    c) The cone is formed by the body of the incus.
    d) The space between the ice cream cone and the scutum is called Prussak's space.
    e) The cone is common involved in Paget's disease.

133. In durul tail sign:
    a) Represents thickening and enhancement of the dura mater in continuity with mass.
    b) Represents reactive changes.
    c) It is due tumour invasion.
    d) Usually multiple.
    e) Should be seen in two successive images through the tumour and it must enhance more the tumour.

134. Which of the following statements are true:
    a) The diameter of the spinal canal at C.5 is 25 mm.
    b) The greatest inter-pedicular distance occurs at D.12/11.
    c) Expiration film of the chest is of no value in a child suspected of having inhaled a foreign body.
    d) Abdominal cocoon sign on CT scan indicating sclerosing encapsulating peritoritis.
    e) Apple core appearance on barium enema indicating carcinoma of the bowel.

135. Which of the following congenital malformation can be diagnosed in the first trimester by ultrasound:
    a) Microcephaly.
    b) Anencephaly.

c) Encephalocele.
d) Meningocele.
e) Acrania.

136. Which are pneumatic bone:
    a) Frontal bone.
    b) Parietal bone.
    c) Maxilla bone.
    d) Sphenoid bone.
    e) Temporal.

137. Which of the following tumours show calcification on CT scan:
    a) Ependymoma.
    b) Medulloblastoma.
    c) Meningioma.
    d) Lymphoma.
    e) Craniophyringioma.

138. Struge-Weber syndrome:
    a) Port wine naevus on the face and/or scalp.
    b) Calcifications in the surface of atrophic brain tissue.
    c) Can be bilateral.
    d) Hemiatrophy of the affected side.
    e) Thinning of the skull vault on the affected side.

139. In middle cerebral artery infarction:
    a) Is the most commonly affected territory in a cerebral infarction.
    b) Ipsilateral hemiparesis.
    c) Hyperdense middle cerebral artery sign is seen immediately and represents direct visualisation of the thromboembolism.
    d) Insular ribbon is affected early.
    e) Hemianopia.

140. Osteopathia striata can be presented with:
    a) Hypertelorism.
    b) Facial palsy.
    c) Life-threatening disease.
    d) Frontal bossing.
    e) Mental retardation.

141. CSF Cisterns and their contents:
    a) Cerebello medullary cistern (cisterna magna) contains the vertebral artery and the origin of the posteroinferior cerebellar artery (PICA).
    b) Cisterna magna contains the ninth (IX), tenth(X), eleventh (XI), and twelfth (XII) cranial nerves.
    c) Pontine cistern contains the sixth nerve (VI) cranial.
    d) Interpeduncular cistern contains the basal vein of Rosenthal and the III cranial nerve.
    e) Superior cistern contains the anterior communicating artery and the A1 and proximal A2 of anterior cerebral artery.

142. Herpes simplex encephalitis:
    a) CT scan may be normal.
    b) Contrast enhancement is uncommon during the first week of the disease.
    c) MRI, T1W may shows only general oedema in affected region.
    d) On MRI, T2W images shows hyperintensity of affected white matter and cortex.
    e) MRI, T2 weighted images is more sensitive than DW1/ADC.

143. Intracranial arteries arising from the internal carotid artery are:
    a) Anterior inferior cerebellar artery.
    b) Superior cerebellar artery.
    c) Anterior choroidal artery.
    d) Ophthalmic artery.
    e) Posterior cerebellar artery.

144. In optic nerve sheath meningioma:
    a) Proptosis is common.
    b) When it bilateral may indicate neurofibromatosis type 2.
    c) Optic nerve tram-track sign indicating glioma.
    d) Calcification is rare.
    e) Premalignant.

145. Fluorosis causes:
    a) Sclerosis of skull.
    b) Synostosis.
    c) Pathological fractures.
    d) Can give rise to a characteristic 'fringed' appearance.
    e) Soft tissue sarcoma.

146. Morquio-Brailsford disease, the following are true:
    a) Platyspondyl.
    b) Epiphyseal fragmentation.
    c) Thin narrow limb bones.
    d) Normal lumbar spine.
    e) Normal hand x-ray.

147. In molar tooth sign:
    a) Superficial inter peduncular fossa.
    b) Cerebral vermis hyperplasia.
    c) Normal appearance of the superior cerebellar peduncles on axial MRI images.
    d) Is pathognomonic of Joubert syndrome.
    e) Microcephaly.

148. Neurofibromatosis can be associated with:
    a) Pheochondromocytoma.
    b) Bilateral gliomata of the optic nerve.
    c) Renal artery aneurysms.
    d) Fibroids in uterus.
    e) Osteomalasia.

149. In chordoma:
    a) Destructive bony tumour.
    b) All are locally malignant tumour.
    c) The two ends of the spinal column are specially affected.
    d) Commonly in young female.
    e) Can produced a large soft tissue mass swelling within the pelvis.

150. In neuroendocrine tumour:
    a) Most commonly occurs in the intestine.
    b) More than 75% of NETs metastasize to the liver.
    c) High specificity of Ga-68 PET/CT.
    d) It is easy to differentiate from multiple haemangioma by CT alone.
    e) Ga-68 PET/CT has a positive predictive value of 100%.

151. Clubfoot (Pes cavus) seen in:
    a) Friedreich's ataxia.
    b) Acromegaly.
    c) Nail-patella syndrome.

d) Amniotic band sequence.
e) Peroneal muscular atrophy.

152. Dense sclerotic vertebra seen in:
    a) Lymphoma.
    b) Paget's disease.
    c) Hurler syndrome.
    d) Myeloma.
    e) Mastocytosis.

153. Squaring of one or more vertebral bodies found in:
    a) Acromegaly.
    b) Alkaptonuria.
    c) Reiter's syndrome.
    d) Rheumatoid arthritis.
    e) Paget's disease.

154. Posterior scalloping of lumbar vertebral bodies is a recognised feature of:
    a) Multiple myeloma.
    b) Spinal haemangioma.
    c) Mucopolysaccharidosis.
    d) Acromegaly.
    e) Achondroplasia.

155. Beaked or hooked-shaped vertebrae seen in:
    a) Cretinism.
    b) Hurler's syndrome (Gargolism).
    c) Phenylketonuria.
    d) Renal osteodystrophy.
    e) Lupus erythematosis.

156. In substernal thyroid:
    a) Characteristically displaces trachea.
    b) Usually project below arch of aorta.
    c) Prolonged enhancement with contrast on CT scan.
    d) Radioisotope scan is diagnostic.
    e) Posterior mediastinum in location.

157. The following statements are true:
   a) Rugger-jersey spine and hyperparathyroidism.
   b) Rigler's sign indicating presence of a pneumoperitonium.
   c) Rachitis rosary and anticonvulsant therapy.
   d) Rice grain calcifications of the soft tissue and haematuria.
   e) Reverse 3 sign and sigmoid valvulus.

158. The following statements are true:
   a) Air crescent sign on CT scan in aspergillomas.
   b) Absent bow-tie sign in bucket handle tears.
   c) Anteater's nose sign in tarsal coalition.
   d) Berry aneurysm and horseshoe kidney.
   e) Blade of grass sign in Garre sclerosing osteomyelitis.

159. An 8-year-old girl with vision loss, café-au-lat skin pigmentation, bowing long bones. The following condition is likely diagnosis:
   a) McCune-Albright syndrome.
   b) Neurofibromatosis.
   c) Osteomalacia.
   d) Osteochondritis.
   e) Renal osteodystrophy.

160. Dysplasia cerebellar gangliocytoma 'Lhermitte-Duclos disease':
   a) Typically presented to raised intracranial pressure.
   b) Arises from the cortex.
   c) Usually bilateral.
   d) Commonly in the 1st decade of life.
   e) Associated with Cowden syndrome.

161. The following statements are true:
   a) The vagus nerve supply the gastrointestinal tract.
   b) The vagus nerve supply the larynx.
   c) Metopic suture persists in adult life in more than 40%.
   d) Foramen routundum of both sides are often asymmetrical.
   e) The base of the skull is formed in membrane.

162. In pituitary microadenoma:
   a) Is less than 40 mm in size.
   b) Contrast enhanced MRI have a sensitivity of 90%.
   c) On T1 MRI usually hyperintense to normal pituitary.

d) Asymptomatic microadenoma is common.
e) Transsphenoidal hypopphysectomy is the treatment of choice.

163. In pituitary macroadenomas:
    a) Most common suprasellar mass in adults.
    b) Is greater than 10 mm in size.
    c) It is approximately twice as common as microadenoma.
    d) Calcification is common.
    e) On MRI is typically hypointense on T1.

164. Expansion of the middle fossa seen in:
    a) Hygroma.
    b) Tubercoloma.
    c) Subarachnoid cyst.
    d) Chronic subdural hematoma.
    e) Hydatid cyst.

165. In Friedreich's ataxia:
    a) Kyphoscoliosis.
    b) Pectus excavatum.
    c) Cerebral atrophy.
    d) Klippel-Feil syndrome.
    e) Pes cavus.

166. The following are components of basal ganglia:
    a) Lentiform nucleus.
    b) Caudate nucleus.
    c) Red nucleus.
    d) Clausstum.
    e) Amygdaloid complex.

167. In cytotoxic cerebral oedema:
    a) Most commonly seen in cerebral ischemia.
    b) Represents the redistribution of water from extracellular to intracellular compartments.
    c) Low signal on ADC.
    d) High signal on DW1.
    e) Enhanced on CT scan.

168. In vasogenic cerebral oedema:
   a) The blood brain barrier is intact.
   b) Mainly affects the grey matter.
   c) It is intracellular oedema.
   d) On CT scan the grey-white matter differentiation is maintained, the oedema extending in finger-like fashion.
   e) MRI shows hyperintense T2 and FLAIR signals which do not show restricted diffusion.

169. In marburg multiple sclerosis:
   a) Only one very large lesion may be present.
   b) Can resemble brain tumour on MRI.
   c) Can resemble brain abscess or on MRI.
   d) MR spectroscopic examination of the perifocal edema shows normal metabolites ratio and peaks.
   e) Decreased lipid/lactose is a feature on MR spectroscopic examination.

170. In mucocele of paranasal sinuses:
   a) Is end stage of chronically obstructed sinus.
   b) May causes unilateral proptosis.
   c) Visual field defect.
   d) Commonly affect the maxillary sinuses.
   e) Hypointense on T1W1 and signal void on T2W1.

171. Abnormal countour of the calvarium seen in:
   a) Sturge-Weber syndrome.
   b) Hyperphosphatasia.
   c) Wilson's disease
   d) Tam-o-shanter skull.
   e) Turner's syndrome.

172. The following lesions can be hypointense in T1 and T2:
   a) Acute haematoma.
   b) Meningioma.
   c) Gliosis.
   d) Calcifications.
   e) Metal.

173. Cerebellopontine angle mass seen in:
    a) Meningioma.
    b) Colloid cyst.
    c) Chordoma.
    d) Epidermoid.
    e) Arachoid cyst.

174. In leptomeningeal cyst:
    a) Usually diagnosed clinically.
    b) History of trauma in children.
    c) Herniation of pia and archoid layers through the dural tear.
    d) Brain is intact.
    e) MRI the cyst isointense with CSF and communicating with subarachnoid space.

175. Abnormal solitary osteolytic skull lesion seen in:
    a) Osteoporosis circumscripta.
    b) Sebaceous cyst.
    c) Osteoma.
    d) Rodent ulcer.
    e) Hydatid cyst.

176. Parasitic disease that gives intracranial calcification.
    a) Cysticercosis.
    b) Paragonimiasis.
    c) Dracunculus medinesis.
    d) Trichinosis.
    e) Hydatid cyst.

177. A 40-year-old female patient presented with recurrent headaches. MRI shows an extra-axial, dural-based, and enhanced lesion. The possible diagnosis:
    a) Glioma.
    b) Meningioma.
    c) Schwannoma.
    d) Arteriovenous malformation.
    e) Pituitary adenoma.

178. The normal lucencies in skull vault are:
    a) Pacchionian impressions.
    b) Vascular impressions.

c) Parietal foramen.
d) Sutural diastasis.
e) Thinning of parietal bone.

179. In colloid cyst:
a) May be presented with thunderclap headache.
b) Is extra ventricular mass of the 3rd ventricle.
c) Located at the foramen of monro.
d) Typically hyperdense on unenhanced CT scan.
e) Typically enhanced on MRI T1 C+.

180. In choroid plexus:
a) Heavy calcification seen in neurofibromatosis.
b) Choroid plexus papilloma is common tumour.
c) Over production of spinal fluid (CSF) in papilloma.
d) Choroid plexus cyst can be bilateral and multiple may cause obstructive hydrocephalus.
e) Choroid plexus cyst is associated with Klinefelter syndrome.

181. In empty sella:
a) Is an empty pituitary fossa.
b) Associated with benign intracranial hypertension.
c) MRI is the modality of choice for confirming the diagnosis.
d) Indistinguishable from those of patients with a pituitary mass on CT scan.
e) Associated with Sheehan's syndrome.

182. White matter changes on MRI seen in:
a) Secondary to shunting.
b) Multiple sclerosis.
c) Multiple infarctions.
d) Adrenal leukodystrophy.
e) Spinocerebellar degeneration.

183. Cerebellar cortical degeneration seen in:
a) Alcoholism.
b) Malignancy.
c) Endocrine disorders.
d) Athletics.
e) Obesity.

184. In brain stone:
    a) Is a cerebral calculus.
    b) Causes hydrocephalus.
    c) Usually multiples.
    d) Due to cysticercosis.
    e) Normal on CT scan.

185. Risk factors of superior sagittal sinus thrombosis are:
    a) Pregnancy.
    b) Dehydration.
    c) Multiple sclerosis.
    d) Hypercoaguable states.
    e) Pancreatitis.

186. Radiographic features of superior sagittal sinus thrombosis:
    a) Cord sign.
    b) Dense vein sign.
    c) Empty delta sign.
    d) Multiploner reformatted CT venography is sensitive in more than 90%.
    e) MR venogram will demonstrate good of flow.

187. In non-odontogenic lucent lesions of the jaw:
    a) Multiple myeloma.
    b) Radicular cyst.
    c) Cherubism.
    d) Ameloblastoma.
    e) Aneurismal bone cyst.

188. In periapical cyst (radicular cysts):
    a) Result from infection of the tooth.
    b) Centred on the apex of the tooth.
    c) Usually about 3 cm in size.
    d) Plain radiograph appear as round or pear-shaped unilocular, lucent lesion in the periapical region.
    e) Usually associated with uncontrolled diabetes.

189. In statue cyst (Lingual salivary gland inclusion defect):
    a) Is a cortical defect near the angle of the mandible.
    b) Contain clear fluid.
    c) Usually discovered by chance during routine dental radiography.

d) It is premalignant.
e) Usually multiple.

190. In ameloblastoma:
    a) Previously known as an adamantinoma of the jaw.
    b) Painless mass near the angle of the mandible.
    c) Presented usually in the 1st decades of life.
    d) Can involve the maxilla.
    e) On CT scan classically seen as a multiloculated expansile 'soap-bubble' lesion with well-demarcated borders.

191. In dentigerous cysyt:
    a) Typically painless.
    b) May be presented as a deep neck abscess.
    c) Commonly involve the mandibular third molar.
    d) On plain radiograph appear as unilocular well-defined pericoronal radiolucencies centred on impacted or unerupted tooth.
    e) Usually multiple.

192. The ventricular system:
    a) Choroid plexus calcification of the fourth ventricle is seen in a good lateral view on plain x-ray occasionally.
    b) CSF is produced at the rate of 500 ml/day.
    c) The ventricles contain about 100 ml of CSF.
    d) Asymmetry of frontal and occipital horns is abnormal.
    e) Dilatation of the temporal horns is a sensitive indicator of hydrocephalus.

193. Cerebellum:
    a) The superior cerebellar peduncle is oriented horizontally.
    b) The superior cerebellar peduncle passes from cerebellum to the pons.
    c) The middle cerebellar peduncles are the largest.
    d) The inferior cerebellum peduncles passes from cerebellum to medulla.
    e) Flocculus of cerebellum enhanced more on contrast administration than the rest of cerebellum.

194. Myelination in T2W images:
    a) The genu of corpus callosum myelinates by 8–11 months.
    b) The frontal white matter is the last to myelinate.
    c) The anterior limb of internal capsule myelinates by 12–14 months.
    d) T2W images are ideal for assessment of myelination after 6 months.
    e) The adult myelination pattern is established by 2 years.

195. Lesions that produce no signal in T1 and T2W MRI images:
    a) Tendon.
    b) High flow.
    c) Gliosis.
    d) Metal.
    e) Chronic haematoma.

196. Myelination of brain:
    a) Inversion recovery images are ideal for assessment of myelination till 2 years of age.
    b) At birth the complete brainstem and cerebellum are myelinated.
    c) The optic radiation is myelinated soon after birth.
    d) The ventral pons is myelinated at 3 months.
    e) The corpus callosum is myelinated at 6 months.

197. Pineal region tumour differential possibilities are:
    a) Osteoma.
    b) Meningioma.
    c) Epidermoid.
    d) Germinoma.
    e) Blastoma.

198. In pineal cyst:
    a) Usually multiple.
    b) Usually symptomatic.
    c) Associates with neurofibromatosis.
    d) Can causing hydrocephalus.
    e) MRI shows higher signal intensity compared to that of CSF in the ventricles.

199. CSF cisterns and their contents:
    a) Cistern magna-posterior inferior cerebellar artery.
    b) Pre-pontine cistern – XI nerve.
    c) Ambient cistern – superior cerebellar arteries.
    d) Interpeduncular cistern – trochlear nerve.
    e) Quadrigeminal cistern – venous confluence.

200. Cranial nerves:
    a) The cranial nerve with the longest intracranial course is abducent nerve.
    b) The vestibulocochlear nerve has hearing role only.
    c) The cranial nerve to show neurobiotaxis is facial nerve.
    d) All the cranial nerves are lined by Schwann cells.
    e) All cranial nerves have sensory and motor components.

201. The pinal gland:
    a) Calcified in 70% of cases on CT scan.
    b) 50% on plain films shows pineal calcification.
    c) Calcification seen from 7 years onwards.
    d) Situated in the anterior aspect of third ventricle.
    e) There are two laminae arising from the pineal gland.

202. The following are normal calcifications in the skull:
    a) Choroid plexus of the 4th ventricle.
    b) Petroclinoid ligament.
    c) Choroid plexus.
    d) Interclinoid ligament.
    e) Hobenular commissure.

203. Skull radiology:
    a) There is no subarachnoid space in the sella.
    b) The arterial impressions are larger than the venous impressions.
    c) The diploic veins have two recognised valves within.
    d) Parietal foramina transmit the emissary vein of santorini.
    e) The posterior cerebral artery is situated against the free edge of falax cerebri.

204. In the intervertebral disc:
    a) The articular plate is a disc of hyaline cartilage.
    b) The annulus fibrosus is attached to edge of the articular plate.

c) The nucleus pulposus is semi gelatinous remnant of the notochord.
d) Spondylosis is commonly due to degenerative ageing process.
e) Schmorl's node is a congenital disc prolapse.

205. The following foramina transmit the corresponding structures:
a) Foramina ovale – accessory meningeal artery.
b) Foramina spinosum – middle meningeal artery.
c) Foramen rotundum – mandibular division of trigeminal nerve.
d) Pterygoid canal – transmits Vidain nerve.
e) Foramen lacerum – transmits the small meningeal branches of the ascending pharyngeal artery.

206. Lesions hyperintense on T1 but hypointense in T2:
a) Meningioma.
b) Thyroid metastasis.
c) Dermoid.
d) Melanoma metastasis.
e) Chronic haematoma.

207. In the spinal cord the following are true:
a) Measures 42–45 cm in length.
b) Is about 1 cm in diameter.
c) Normally ends at the level of L3/L4 vertebra.
d) Diastematomyelia is reduplication of the cord.
e) In dysraphism the conus medullaris is attached to the coccyx.

208. The skull:
a) Made up of 5 bones.
b) The base is formed in membrane.
c) Venous lacunate are most common in the occipital bone adjacent to the transverse sinus.
d) Metopic suture persists in adult in more than 40%.
e) Foramen rotundum of both sides are often asymmetrical.

209. Arachnoid cap cells are seen:
a) Root sleeves of spinal nerves.
b) Root sleeves of cranial nerves.
c) Veins.
d) Choroid plexus.
e) Adjacent to the superior sagittal sinus.

210. Structures enhancing on contrast administration in CT:
   a) Dura matter.
   b) Pituitary.
   c) Choroid plexus.
   d) Pinal gland.
   e) Infundibulum.

211. Lesions hyperintense on T1 and T2W:
   a) Subacute haematoma.
   b) Melanoma.
   c) Cholesteatoma.
   d) Posterior pituitary.
   e) Flowing blood.

212. MRI scan of brain:
   a) The grey matter is hyperintense to white matter in proton density images.
   b) The white matter appears bright in T2 and dark in T1.
   c) The grey matter appears dark on T2 and bright on T1.
   d) Internal capsule is bright on T2.
   e) The globus pallidus and substantia nigra are bright in T1 and dark in T2.

213. CT and MRI of brain:
   a) The normal CT scans images are parallel to the line tangential to orbital roof.
   b) The white matter appears brighter than the grey matter in CT scans of the brain.
   c) Choroid plexus is hyperintense in unenhanced MR images.
   d) Images of skull base are taken parallel to the line passing to from posterior lip of foramen magnum.
   e) The midline and posterior fossa are best evaluated by CT scan.

214. The following structures enhance on Gadelinium administration:
   a) Dura matter.
   b) Pituitary gland.
   c) Choroid plexus of 4th ventricle.
   d) Transverse sinus.
   e) Cavernous sinus.

215. The skull and sutures:
    a) Anterior fontanelle closes in the first year.
    b) The lambda suture closes by the second month.
    c) The pterion closes in the 9 months.
    d) The metopic suture closes at 5 years.
    e) Diploic veins are present at birth.

216. The following components of basal ganglia:
    a) Lentiform nucleus.
    b) Caudate nucleus.
    c) Red nucleus.
    d) Amygdala.
    e) Clausstum.

217. In pituitary gland:
    a) The infundibulum is larger in male.
    b) The infundibulum is enlarged if it is larger than the basilar artery.
    c) The gland in uniformly hypointense in neonate.
    d) The anterior and the posterior lobes of the pituitary gland can't be separately identified in MR scan.
    e) The posterior pituitary normally shows high signal in T1W1.

218. In Susac syndrome (retinocochleocerebral vasculapathy):
    a) Usually affects young women.
    b) Classical clinical triad of bilateral hearing loss, branch retinal artery occlusion, and encephalopathy.
    c) MRI feature are T2 hyperintense lesions are rounded and located in the middle layers of the body and splenium of the corpus callosum.
    d) Multiple lesions are commonly at periventricular in location.
    e) Acute lesions may show restricted diffusion and contrast enhancement.

219. Hyperextension C2 fracture:
    a) Cord compression is rare.
    b) Commonly diagnosed on radiographs.
    c) Vascular compromise can cause central cord syndrome.
    d) Associated with fracture mandible.
    e) The classic findings associated with this injury are prevertebral soft tissue swelling.

1. a. True   b. True   c. False   d. True   e. True

Homonymous hemianopia can be congenital, but usually caused by brain injury such as from stroke, trauma, tumours infection, demyelination, or following surgery.

2. a. False   b. False   c. False   d. True   e. True

Lacunar Skull / Luckenschadel Skull
- Bone dysplasia of skull consisting of multiple oval lucencies separated by dense, bony ridges.
- Associated with
    o   Neural tube defects, especially myelomeningocele.
    o   Chiari II malformation.
    o   Encephalocele.
- Inner table more affected than outer.
- Present at birth.
- Unrelated to increase intracranial pressure.
- Lacunae are bounded by normally ossified bone.
- Most prominent in parietal bones.
- Small posterior fossa associated with Chiari II malformation.
- Normal convolutional markings associated with synostosis at an older age.
- Appearance resolves spontaneously by age 6 months.

3. a. True   b. True   c. False   d. True   e. True

Bony sclerosis of the base of the skull may be associated with basilar impression.

There are many causes some are not homogeneously sclerosed.

Any weakness of the bones may give rise to invagination of the base of the skull, e.g. any cause of osteoporosis or osteomalacia.

Other causes congenital e.g. atlanto-occipital fusion, Klipple-feil deformity or stenosis of foramen magnum, Achondroplasia aqueduet stenosis, cleidocranial dysplasia, osteopetrosis.

Collagen disease e.g. rheumatoid arthritis, ankylosing spondylitis.

Trauma and infection including tuberculosis others e. g. Paget's disease, mucopolysaccharidosis, histocytosis X.

Collagen disease, e.g., rheumatoid arthritis, ankylosing spondylitis.

Trauma and infection including tuberculosis others, e.g., Paget's disease, mucopolysaccharidosis, histocytosis X.

4.   a. True   b. True   c. False   d. True   e. False

Juvenile angiofibroma is a common benign nasopharyngeal tumour. Can grow to enormous size and locally invade vital structures.

Mean age is 15 years, almost exclusively in males. Recurrent severe epistaxis (59%). Nasal speech due to nasal obstruction (11%). Invasion of sphenoid sinus.

Widening of pterygopalatine fossa (90%).

On MR, there is intermediate signal intensity on T1W1 with discrete punctuate areas of hypo intensity (secondary to highly vascular stroma).

5.   a. True   b. True   c. False   d. True   e. False

Rubella (German measles) – infants (in uterotransmission) neonatal dwarfism, retinopathy, cataracts, deafness, mental deficiency. No periosteal reactin or spina bifida.

6. a. False   b. True   c. True   d. True   e. True

Cranial nerve palsy – any variety of a tonal muscular conditions characterised parts as the hands, arms, or legs or of entire body.

7. a. False   b. False   c. False   d. False   e. True

Ranula is mucus retention cyst that occurs in the sublingual gland that does not communicate with the duct. It may be due to prior surgery or obstruction of the sublingual gland or its duct. It is either simple (true cyst) or plunging (deep). It is a pseudocysts extended below the level of the mylohyoid.

Typical CT findings include smooth well-delineated, cystic mass with no enhancing wall. Unless if infected (in distinguished from abscess) on MRI shows low signal intensity on T1W1 and high signal intensity on T2W1 however vary with protein content.

8. a. True   b. True   c. True   d. False   e. True

Paraspinal Soft Tissue Mass
- Aortic aneurysm, tortuous aorta.
- Hematoma, traumatic, or spontaneous.
- Lymphoma.
- Metastatic neoplasm.
- Myeloma.
- Neurogenic tumour (neurofibroma, neurilemmoma, gangioneuron, neuroblastoma).
- Osteoarthritis (spondylosis deformans).
- Osteomyelitis of spine with abscess (e.g., tuberculosis, sarcoid, brucellar, other bacterial).
- Pleural effusion (loculated).
- Bronchogenic cyst.
- Chemodectoma.
- Dilated azygos system (e.g., superior of inferior vena cava obstructed mediastinal varices).
- Eosiphillic granuloma of vertebra.
- Extramedullary haematopoiesis (esp. in thalassemia).
- Intraspinal tumour of hourglass type.
- Mesothelioma.
- Neurenteric cyst.

- Paget's disease (uncalcified osteoid).
- Spine neoplasm, primary (e.g., giant cell tumour, chordoma, sarcoid).

9.   a. True   b. True   c. True   d. True   e. False

A defect in the posterior neural arch commonly seen in the lower lumbar spine, or upper sacral, and nearly associated with neurologic defect seen as isolated anomaly, however, it may be seen in Lipomeningocele, dermoid, epidermoid cyst, and others. It differs from spina bifida aperta being that aperta is always associated with neurologic defect where the posterior element of the vertebra is not fused completely and overlying soft tissue. Seen in meningocele, meningomyelocele, myeloschiasis, myelocystocele.

10.   a. True   b. True   c. True   d. True   e. False

Truncal Vagotomy is a treatment option for chronic duodenal ulcers. Also used in the treatment of obesity. May follow a dysphagia which occurring 7–10 days after operation usually lasts from one to several weeks and resolves spontaneously. The end of the oesophagus is tapering similar to achalasia, this is also atemporarily with time. The stomach is dilated with delay emptying postural hypotension also happen. There are no cardiac arrhythmias.

11.   a. True   b. True   c. False   d. True   e. False

Neuroblastoma is a common solid abdominal mass of infancy, and 3rd most common malignant tumour in infancy (often leukaemia + CNS tumour) and 2nd most common tumour in childhood (often Wilm's tumour). Occasionally present at birth. The tumour origin from the neural crest be anywhere in the sympathetic neural chain. The tumour displace the kidney, abdominal, calcification is common. Increase catecholamine production. Intractable diarrhoea due to increase in vasoactive intestinal polypeptides (VIP). The pelvis involves 5% (organ of Zuckerkandle).

12.   a. True   b. False   c. False   d. True   e. True

Tullio's phenomenon is momentary vertigo caused by loud, notably occurring in case of active labyrinthine fistula.

Superior Semicircular Canal Dehiscence Syndrome (SSCDS) can be confirmed by thin-section CT or Digital Volume Tomography (DVT).

Perilymphatic fistula, disruption of labyrinthine bone due to chronic otitis media can cause similar symptoms as in SSCDS.

SSCDS mostly unilateral and presents a normal finding without any symptoms in up to 4% of adults and up to 14% of children. Onset of symptoms is typically in adulthood usually between 30 and 50 years old. This is non-metabolic or iatrogenic condition. It may be congenital or inflammatory.

13. a. False   b. True   c. True   d. False   e. True

Intracranial or intra-orbital tumours are present in neurofibromatosis (central form) optic nerve glioma, manifest at CT scan as fusiform but often rather bulbous widening and increase attenuation of the intra-orbital portion of the nerve with homogeneous enhancement after IV > contrast medium. Intracranial extension manifest as peduncular fossa is a grave prognostic sign.

Optic nerve sheath meningioma is rare tumours but show an increase incidence in neurofibromatosis.

14. a. False   b. True   c. False   d. True   e. False

Subarachnoid Haemorrhage (SAH)
- Bleeding into the subarachnoid space, between the pia mater and the arachnoid.
- Most common causes are rupture of an intracranial aneurysm or head trauma also seen in arteriovenous malformation (AVM), extension from intracerebral haemorrhage, arteriovenous fistulae, meningitis, and neoplasm.

Clinical Findings
- Headache is most common symptom, nausea, vomiting, and confusion.

Imaging Findings
- Unenhanced CT of the brain is the study of choice for establishing presence of SAH.
- CT angiography and MRA have replaced conventional angiography in most institutions for the identification and location of the aneurysm itself.

- Acute haemorrhage appears as high-attenuation (white) material that fills the normally black subarachnoid spaces.
- Over the convexities of the brain, SAH produces white, branching densities representing the normally black sulci filled with blood.
- From communicating hydrocephalus is seen in subacute period.
- MR angiography is useful in identifying the location of aneurysms.
- SAH from an arteriovenous malformation has a better prognosis than SAH from a ruptured aneurysm.

15. a. True   b. True   c. True   d. True   e. False

16. a. True   b. True   c. False   d. False   e. True

17. a. True   b. True   c. False   d. True   e. True

18. a. True   b. True   c. True   d. False   e. True

19. a. True   b. True   c. True   d. False   e. False

20. a. True   b. False   c. True   d. False   e. false

21. a. True   b. True   c. True   d. False   e. False

22. a. True   b. True   c. True   d. False   e. True

23. a. True   b. True   c. True   d. True   e. False

24. a. True   b. True   c. True   d. False   e. False

25. a. True   b. False   c. True   d. True   e. False

26. a. True   b. True   c. True   d. False   e. True

27. a. True   b. True   c. False   d. False   e. True

28. a. True   b. True   c. True   d. False   e. False

29. a. False b. True   c. True   d. True   e. True

30. a. False b. False   c. True   d. True   e. True

31.	a. False	b. True	c. True	d. True	e. True
32.	a. False	b. False	c. True	d. True	e. True
33.	a. True	b. True	c. True	d. True	e. False
34.	a. True	b. True	c. True	d. False	e. False
35.	a. True	b. False	c. True	d. True	e. False
36.	a. True	b. True	c. True	d. False	e. False
37.	a. True	b. False	c. False	d. True	e. True
38.	a. True	b. True	c. True	d. True	e. False
39.	a. True	b. True	c. False	d. False	e. True
40.	a. True	b. True	c. True	d. False	e. True
41.	a. True	b. True	c. True	d. False	e. True
42.	a. True	b. False	c. True	d. False	e. True
43.	a. True	b. False	c. True	d. True	e. True
44.	a. False	b. True	c. True	d. True	e. True
45.	a. False	b. False	c. True	d. False	e. True
46.	a. True	b. True	c. True	d. False	e. True
47.	a. False	b. True	c. True	d. True	e. True
48.	a. True	b. True	c. False	d. True	e. True
49.	a. False	b. True	c. True	d. False	e. True
50.	a. True	b. True	c. True	d. False	e. True
51.	a. True	b. True	c. True	d. False	e. False

52.	a. False	b. True	c. False	d. True	e. False
53.	a. True	b. True	c. True	d. False	e. True
54.	a. True	b. True	c. True	d. False	e. True
55.	a. True	b. False	c. True	d. False	e. False
56.	a. False	b. True	c. True	d. False	e. True
57.	a. True	b. True	c. True	d. False	e. True
58.	a. True	b. True	c. True	d. True	e. False
59.	a. True	b. True	c. True	d. True	e. False
60.	a. True	b. True	c. False	d. True	e. True
61.	a. True	b. False	c. True	d. True	e. False

Also seen in brain tumour, hydrocephalus meningitis, hypervitaminosis A as well as hypovitaminosis A, leukaemia, lymphoma, increase intracranial pressure, etc.

62.	a. False	b. False	c. True	d. True	e. True
63.	a. True	b. True	c. True	d. False	e. True
64.	a. True	b. True	c. True	d. True	e. False
65.	a. True	b. True	c. False	d. True	e. True
66.	a. True	b. True	c. False	d. True	e. False
67.	a. False	b. True	c. False	d. False	e. True
68.	a. True	b. True	c. False	d. True	e. True
69.	a. True	b. False	c. True	d. False	e. False
70.	a. True	b. True	c. True	d. False	e. False

71. a. True   b. True   c. True   d. False   e. False

72. a. True   b. True   c. True   d. False   e. False

73. a. False   b. True   c. True   d. False. False

74. a. False   b. True   c. True   d. False   e. False

In generalised convulsion following injection of contrast medium should be treated by:
- Calcium Gluconate IV in treatment of hypocalcemia tetany. 100–300 mg elemental IV over 5–10 minutes followed by continuous IV infusion at 0.5 mg/kg/hr.
- Adrenaline is epinephrine. A hormone that is secreted by the adrenal medulla in response to stress and increases heart rate, pulse rate, blood pressure, and rises the level of glucose and lipids.
- Coramine is nikethamide is a stimulant that mainly affects the respiratory cycle. It was used in the mid-twentieth century.
- Pentothal (Thiopental sodium) as a sole anesthetic agent for brief (15 min.) procedures.

75. a. True   b. True   c. False   d. True   e. False

Laryngeal Papillomas / Reccurrent Respiratory Papillomatosis
- Most common benign tumour of the trachea in children (60% of all benign tumours).
- 2nd most common benign tumour of trachea in adults. Majority of primary tracheal tumours are malignant. In over 80% of cases, multiple papillomas occur in the trachea.
- Tracheal papillomas is associated with a laryngeal papilloma in 36%.
- Because of its high occurrence rate, it is also called Recurrent Respiratory Papillomatosis (RRP).
- Most common in children and then again 20–40 years of age.
- Children usually present around age 2–3 years. Cough, hacking in nature, audible wheezing, haemoptysis, stridor, dysphagia, pneumonia, and aphonia.
- Adult-onset disease. Less severe than juvenile form. Male:female ratio in adults is 4:1. Painless hoarseness.
- Diagnosis is made using flexible fiberoptic laryngoscopy.

- Chest radiograpghs are usually normal. Papillomas can present as multiple nodules in the chest, some of which may cavitate.
- CT scans of the neck and chest will demonstrate the extent of the lesions.

76. a. True   b. False   c. False   d. True   e. False

Pelvic Rhabdomyosarcoma (Botryoid Tumour / Sarcoma Tryoides)
- GU rhabdomyosarcoma originating from any of the pelvis organs.
- Most common location is head and neck. GU is second most common, can originate from bladder, vagina, uterus, prostate, paratesticular tissue, pelvic side walls.
- Peak incidence: 2–6 years old.
- Tumours spread by local extension via lymphatic and haematogenous metastasis to lungs, liver, bones.
- On CT, heterogenous enhancing mass.
- On MRI, signal intensity between muscle and fat, enhances with gadolinium.
- Bone scan to evaluate bony metastatic disease.

77. a. True   b. True   c. True   d. False   e. True

Mucocele of Frontal Sinuses
- True cystic lesion lines by sinus mucosa.
- Mucocele occurs as a result of complete obstruction of sinus ostium. The body walls of the sinus are remodelled as the pressure of secretions increases.
- Location – frontal 65%, ethmoidal 25%, maxillary less than 10%, sphenoid (rare), pyelocele (infected mucocele).
- Typical isodense by CT scan.
- MRI signal intensity.
  - Low T1, high T2 – serious content
  - High T1, high T2 – high protein content
  - Low T1, low T2 – viscous content
- Some local causes of hypertelovism are fibrous dysplasia, leontiasis ossea, midline dermoid or teratoma, cranium bifidum, and others.

78. a. True   b. False   c. False   d. False   e. False

Microcephaly
- The head circumference below the normal range. May be associated with mental retardation.

Main Causes:
1. Intrauterine infection (toxoplasmosis, rubella, CMB, herpes syphilis)
2. Toxic agents, e.g., drugs, hypoxia, radiation, maternal phenylketonuria
3. Premature craniosynostosis
4. Chromosomal abnormalities
5. Meckel-Gruber syndrome

79. a. True   b. False   c. True   d. False   e. True

Widened Interpedicular Distance in the Lumbar Region
- The tranverse distance between the centre of the two pedicale in the same vertebra can be short, e.g., in Achondroplasia or wide in mucopolysarcoidosis.
- Diastomatomyelinia (is a linear vertical division or reduplication of the spinal cord in the midline). The lower thoracic and upper lumbar areas as the most common sites. This part of the cord of ten transfixed by bony or fibrous ridge or spicule extending from the vertebral body infront to the dura behind the cord.
- The spinal canal is widened over several segments. The interpedicular distance is increased however the pedicles are not eroded.
- Jone-Thomson ratio between 0.5 and 0.22 less than 0.22 indicate spinal stenosis (width of spinal canal multiply by height divided over height and width of the vertebral body of the same).

80. a. False   b. False   c. True   d. False   e. True

Brucellosis (Mediterranean Fever) / Malta Fever / Gastric Remittent Fever / Undulant Fever

Brucella organisms is gram-negative. The sequelae are highly variable and may include granulomatous hepatitis, spondylitis, anaemia, leucopenia, thrombocytopenia, meningitis, uveitis, optic neurosis, endocarditis, arthritis (but not hypertrophic osteoarthropathy.

81. a. True   b. True   c. False   d. True   e. True

Calcification in the orbits may occur in many conditions particularly in cataract, foreign body. Phlebolith (e.g., orbital varices, haemangioma) phytosis bulbi (old trauma or infection of ethmoid or vitreous with shrunked globe). Retiroblastoma, aneurysm, or atherosclerosis of internal carotid artery ans or ophthalmic artery.

Sarcoidosis, syphilis, diabetes, collagen disease (e.g., band keratopathy of cornea in rheumatoid arthritis). Hematoma, myositic ossificans of extra-ocular muscles; hypercalcemia (metastatic calcification in hypervitaminosis D, primary and secondary hyperparathyroidism, multiple myeloma, milk-alkali syndrome).

Idiopathic; intraocular infection, e.g., abscess, TB, intracranial neoplasm, e.g., meningioma, dermoid cyst, optic glioma. Plexiform neurofibroma, lacrimal gland carcinoma, haemangioendothelioma, mucocele invading the orbit.

82. a. True   b. True   c. True   d. False   e. True

Lemierre Syndrome (Necrobacillosis)
Lemierre syndrome – infection of the parapharyngeal space spread to carotid space, where it can result in ipsilateral jugular venous thrombosis.

Pulmonary septic emboli is very common, initially patient present with acute pharyngitis, followed by fever, rigors, tenderness, swelling, and pain over the angle of the jaw may also be present.

By contrast, enhanced CT scan is the imaging study of choice in finding the inciting abscess, distended veins, intraluminal filling defects, enhancing walls of veins.

Treated by antibiotic and/or anticoagulation.

83. a. False   b. True   c. True   d. False   e. True

Hygroma (Lymphangioma)
- Cystic lymphangioma, single or multiloculated fluid-filled cavities on either side if fetal neck, head, or trunk.

- Associated with chromosomal abnormalities in about 70%, e.g., Turner syndrome, Noonan's syndrome.
- It can be subdural in location. The CSF-fluid collection within subdural space that appear as isointense to CSF/hyperintense to CSF on T1W1 (increase protein content).
- Radioluscent crescent-shaped collection as in acute subdural hematoma on CT scan.

84. a. True   b. False   c. True   d. True   e. False

Vein Galen Malformation (Vein of Galen Aneurysm / Misnomer)
- Is intracranial arteriovenous malformation involving aneurismal dilatation of the vein of Galen.
- Most common extra cardiac cause of high-output congestive heart failure in neonatal period.
- Large extracardiac left to right shunt.
- Patient is acyanotic cardiomegaly, increased pulmonary vascularity, pulmonary oedema.
- Cranial color Doppler ultrasonography shown.
- Aneurymally dilated vein of Galen.
- T1W1 MRI depicts flow void in aneurysm compressing aqueduct, leading to hydrocephalus.
- On echocardiography, retrograde diastolic flow in descending aorta due to steal phenomenon. Dilated central veins with abnormally pulsatile flow signal. Dilated ascending aorta and its branches (carotid and vertebral arteries). Global cardiac enlargement.

85. a. False   b. False   c. False   d. False   e. True

Bone Tumours Involving Vertebral Bodies
- Tumour of the vertebra may be expansile, e.g., multiple myeloma, plasmocytoma, metastasis, Paget's disease, eosinophilic granuloma.
- May be expansile solitary or multiple, some are benign, e.g., osteochondroma, osteoblastoma, osteoid osteoma, aneurismal bone cyst, some are malignant, e.g., chondroma, plasmocytoma, angiosarcoma, Ewing tumour, lymphoma.
- Some bony tumours favouring vertebral bodies, e.g., chordoma, aneurismal bone cyst, leukaemia, lymphoma, haemangioma, osteoid osteoma, osteoblastoma, myeloma, metastasis, eosinophilic granuloma.

86. a. True   b. True   c. True   d. True   e. False

Langerhan's Cell Histocytosis (Eosophilic granuloma, Histocytosis X)
- Idiopathic disorder that can manifest as focal localised or systemic diaease, monostatic involvement > multifocal involvement. Any bone can involve mainly skull, rib, femur as lucent or sclerotic, permeative or geographic well-defined sclerotic or poorly defined borders.
- The edge of the skull lesion described as 'bevelled' inner table involved > outer table.
- Sclerotic rim during healing phase.
- Coalescence of lesions, geographic skull.
- Types: Letterer-Siwe, hand Schueller Christian, Eosinophilic granuloma
- Clinical presentation:
  - Age 2–30 years
  - Mean age 5–10 years
  - Male:female – 2:1
  - Commonly white people, local pain, tenderness, swelling/soft tissue mass, fever, leukocytesis.
- May be treated by excision and curettage, radiation.

87. a. True   b. True   c. True   d. False   e. False

Moya-moya Idiopathic Progressive Arteriopathy of Childhood is progressive narrowing of distal ICA and proximal circle of willis(cow) vessels with secondary collateralization.

Initially described in Japanese children (still more common).

Increase incidence of stroke, intracranial haemorrhage in adults, sudden hemiplegia in children or adolescence.

CT findings show atrophy, intracranial haemorrhage, enhanced dots in basal ganglia.

MRI shows multiple dark dots in basal ganglia on T1W1. There is high signal from small vessel infarcts in cortex and white matter.

The MRA shows narrowing of distal ICA and proximal cow vessels.

88. a. False   b. True   c. True   d. True   e. True

Fibromuscualar Dysplasia (Hyperplasia)
- Female to male ratio 3:1
- Presenting age 25–50 years
- Medial fibroplasias most common
- Renovascular hypertension (if bilateral renal arteries involved)
- Transient ischemic attack
- Intracranial aneurysm/thromboembolic stroke
- Often asymptomatic
- Renal arteries 85% – only 40% have bilateral renal artery involvement
- Less commonly affected: internal carotid (often bilateral), vertebral, mesenteric, celiac, hepatic, iliac arteries.
- If fibromuscular dysplasia is found at any location, one must evaluate carotid arteries for lesions—narrowing of the affected vessel with a 'string of beads' or nodular appearance, due to focal annular repetitive intimal and medial proliferative changes.
- Angioplasty is less invasive and cure rate is approximately 50%.
- Angioplasty suitable for noncalcified short segments.

89. a. True   b. True   c. True   d. True   e. False

Dislocation of the Mandible
- Dislocations of the mandible tend to be uncomfortable but not severely painful for the patient.
    - The presence of a fracture increases the pain.
- Patients are unable to close mouth completely.
- Difficulty speaking and, possibly, swallowing.
- Dislocations may be unilateral or bilateral.
    - Prognathic appearance to jaw when both are dislocated.
- Predisposing conditions.
    - Shallow mandibular fossa may predispose to dislocation.
    - Connective tissue diseases like Marfan's or Echlers-Danlos may have increased risk.
    - Those with previous dislocations are at much greater risk for repeat dislocation.
        - May eventually result in osteoarthritis in TM joint.
- Most dislocations occur spontaneously on opening the mouth widely from yawn, dental work, during seizure.
- Trauma may also produce dislocation.

- o   Trauma involves a downward force on partially opened jaw.
- Normally, the mandibular condyle lies in the mandibular fossa of the temporal bone when the mouth is closed and moves forward slightly when the mouth is open.
- When dislocated, mandibular condyle moves forward and lies anterior to the articular eminence that prevents to the mandibular fossa of the temporal bone.

90. a. False   b. False   c. True   d. True   e. True

Haemangioma of the Spine

General Considerations
- Benign
- Most often located in the lower thoracic, upper lumbar spine
  - o   Skull is second most common location (spoke-wheel appearance)
- Mostly asymptomatic
- More frequent in females
- Peak incidence in 40s
- Multiple in up to 1/3 of cases
- Most often occur in the medullary of bone
- Microscopically, there hamartomatous proliferation of vascular tissue
  - o   Classified as to cavernous, capillary, anteriovenous and venous
  - o   Spine haemangiomas are usually capillary type; skull are cavernous

Clinical Findings
- Usually asymptomatic
- Very slow growing
- No known malignant potential
- Over 40, patients may present with pain from compression fracture

Imaging Findings
- Conventional radiography is usually the first means of imaging haemangiomas
  - o   Prominent trabecular pattern from resorption of trabeculae by enlarged vascular channels produces
    - ▪ Ventricle striations

- o Overall density of vertebral body is increased
- o Cortex is not thickened and vertebral body is not increased in size
- o Small haemangiomas will not be visible on conventional radiographs
- CT
  - o Corduroy (aka accordion, honeycomb, polka-dot) spine from coarse trabeculae seen in cross section
    - Thickened vertebral trabeculae produce a polka-dot appearance
  - o Bone destruction and soft tissue extension may be present but are rare
- MRI
  - o Allows for diagnosis of soft-tissue extension
  - o Increased signal intensity on both T1 (high fate content) and T2 (increased vascularity)
- Nuclear medicine
  - o Usually normal uptake on bone scan

Complications
- Pathologic fracture
- Haemorrhage, when it occurs, is usually iatrogenic
- Thrombosis
- Displacement of adjacent nerves producing pain

91. a. True   b. False   c. False   d. True   e. False

Retropharyngeal Abscess
Pyogenic infection of the retropharyngeal space.

Widening of the retropharyngeal soft tissues following pharyngitis or upper respiratory tract infection, sudden onset of fever, stiff neck, dyspnea, stridor.

Typical age: 6–12 months.

Gas within soft tissues diagnostic of abscess.

CT performed to define extent of disease and help predict causes in which a drainable fluid collection is present.

92. a. True   b. True   c. True   d. False   e. True

Epiglottitis
- Airway obstruction secondary to infectious inflammation of the epiglottis and surrounding tissues.
- On lateral radiograph shows enlargement of the epiglottis and thickening of the epiglottis folds.
- This is life-threatening disease often requiring emergency intubation, mean age 3–5 years.
- Most causes are secondary to hemophilus influenza.
- Much less common causes in group A streptococcus. It may be due to caustic ingestion or bee stings, angioneurotic edema or trauma.

93. a. True   b. True   c. False   d. False   e. True

Enlarged Tonsils
- Enlargement of the adenoid and palatine tonsils in leading cause of obstructive sleep apnea in children.
- It pays a major contributor to childhood learning disabilities such as attention deficit disorder.
- On the lateral radiograph the size of the adenoid greater than 12 mm should be considered abnormal. However adenoids rarely visible radiographically less than 6 months.
- Peak size between 2 and 10 years of age.
- The size begins to decrease during second decade. Enlarged paltine tonsils as prominent soft tissue mass overlying posterior inferior aspect of soft palate. Tonsils may be enlarged in lymphoma.

94. a. False   b. True   c. True   d. False   e. True

Floating Teeth (Loose Teeth)
- Seen in histocytosis X, periodonitis, agranulocytosia, cyclic neutropenia, ameloblastoma, Ewing's sarcoma, familial dyproteinemia, fibrous dysplasia, hyperparathyroidism, hypophosphatasia, leukaemia, lymphoma, Burkitts tumour, melanotic prognoma, acrodynia (mercury) poisoning, metastatic neoplasm (esp. neuroblastoma, retinoblastoma), Papillon-LeFevre syndrome (juvenile periodontosis) plasmacytoma.
- Papillon-LeFevre syndrome is severe destruction of periodontium results in loss of most primary teeth by the age of 4 years associated with hyperkeratosis of psalms and soles of feet.

95. a. True   b. True   c. True   d. True   e. False

Craniosynostosis
- Is premature fusion of one or more of the cranium sutures.
- More often is secondary from failure of growth of the brain.
- Sagittal suture is affected most commonly 50–60%.
- Early fusion of the metopic suture lead to trigonocephaly.
- Early fusion of the sagittal suture give snope of scaphocephaly.
- Brachycephaly is due to early fusion of both coronal sutures.

96. a. True   b. True   c. False   d. False   e. True

Paranasal Osteoma
- Most common tumour of the paranasal sinuses.
- Most frequently seen in the frontal and ethmoid sinuses.
- Benign tumour of membranous bone consisting of dense, compact bone.
- In the skull, they usually arise from the outer table.
- Rarely, large osteoma in the frontal or ethmoid region may displace globe forward and cause proptosis.
- Obstruction of a sinus ostium may lead to infection or formation of a mucocele.
- Very rarely, an osteoma may erode through the dura leading to cerebrospinal fluid Rhinorrhea or intracranial infection.

Imaging Findings
- Well-circumscribed, sharply-marginated round and very dense lesions usually less than 2 cm in size.
- Multiple paranasal osteomas are found in Gardener's syndrome.
- Multiple osteoma of the mandible and maxilla, along with the frontal, sphenoid, and ethmoid sinuses, rarely the long bones or phalanges.
- Cutaneous and soft tissue tumours.
- Association between colonic polyps with a predilection to malignant degeneration.

97. a. False   b. False   c. False   d. False   e. True

Sialolithiasis (Stone in Wharton's or Stensen's duct)
- Most common disease of salivary glands.
- Twice as common in males as females.

- 80–95% occur in submandibular gland or Wharton's duct.
- Stones are most common cause of acute and chronic infection of salivary glands.
- 80% of submandibular stones are opaque; 60% of parotid are opaque
    - Consist of mainly calcium phosphate – not associated with systemic calcium abnormalities.
    - Pain swelling of involved gland – Sialolithiasis cause pain and swelling of the involved salivary gland by obstructing the food-related flow of salivary secretions. Calculi may cause stasis of saliva facilitating bacterial ascentinto the gland and subsequent infection. Some may be asymptomatic.
    - Plain radiography – opaque stone in course of Wharton's (submandibular) or Stensen's Parotid) ducts.
    - CT – stone in duct. Ductal dilatation.
    - MR – inflammation of the gland.
    - Sialography is contraindicated in acute infection or in a patient with a significant contrast allergy.

Treatment
- Conservative
- Surgical removal
- Lithotripsy

98. a. False   b. True   c. False   d. False   e. True

Some causes of multiple intracranial calcification Struge-Weber syndrome, basal cell nevus syndrome, Hypoparathyroidism, pseudohypoparathyroidism, Fahr's disease.

Carbon monoxide intoxication, cytomegalic inclusive disease, encephalitis (e.g., measles, chickenpox, neonatal herpes simplex), hematoma, hypervitaminosis D, hyperparathyroidism, parasitic disease, e.g., cysticercosis, trichinosis, hydatoid cyst.

Toxoplasmosis, tuberculosis, tuberous sclerosis, tumours, Wilson's disease others.

99. a. True   b. False   c. True   d. False   e. True

The sinuses size may be large or small, may be deformed.
- The frontal sinus height – 1.5-2 cm
- The sphenoid sinus width – 1-1.4 cm
- The maxillary sinuses width – 2 cm, height 2 cm

100. a. True   b. True   c. False   d. True   e. True

Thyroid Opthalmopathy
• Patients are usually hyperthyroid but may be euthyroid.
• Usually bilateral thick inferior rectus and medial rectus muscles.
• Seen in diffuse toxic goiter (Grave's disease).

101. a. False   b. False   c. False   d. True   e. True

102. a. True   b. True   c. True   d. False   e. True

Extramedullary Haematopoiesis in Thalassemia
• Response to insufficient blood cell production by production of blood elements outside of the marrow cavity.
• Due to haemolytic anaemias such as sickle cell anaemia, thalassemia, and hereditary sphenocytosis.
• Also seen in prolong iron deficiency anaemia, myelofibrosis and sclerosis, polycythemia, leukaemia, and lymphoma.

103. a. False   b. True   c. True   d. True   e. True

- Also associated with pancreatitis, hepatic steatosis, Friedreich's ataxia, fetal alcohol syndrome.

104. a. True   b. True   c. True   d. False   e. True

105. a. True   b. True   c. False   d. True   e. True

Posterior plagiocephaly is due to lambdoid is fused early in childhood. The anterior plagiocephaly is due one coronal suture fusion early.

106. a. True   b. True   c. False   d. True   e. True

Arnold-Chiari malformation is structural defect in the cerebellum. Affected females are more often than males. May be asymptomatic, others may have symptoms, e.g., headache, vision problems, numbness, muscle weakness problems with balance and coordination and there are 4 types. May be associated with hydrocephalus, spina bifida, synringomyelia, tethered cord syndrome, scoliosis, kyphosis, and others.

107. a. True   b. True   c. False   d. True   e. True

108. a. True   b. True   c. False   d. False e. False

109. a. True   b. True c. False   d. True   e. True

Vertebral pneumatocysts, air-filled cavities within the vertebral bodies similar to other intraosseous pneumatocysts seen elsewhere especially adjacent to the sacroiliac joints. CT scan is diagnostic.

110. a. False b. False c. False d. True   e. False

Hypoxic-ischemic brain injury occurs at any age. Older children near drowning and asphyxiation remain common causes in adult more often a result of cardiac arrest or cerebrovascular disease.

Primarily affects the grey matters structures on CT scan, diffuse oedema with effacement of CSF-containing spaces.

Loss of the candate head density.

111. a. True   b. True   c. True   d. False e. True

Wernicke-Korsakoff syndrome due to thiamine (vitamin B1) deficiency typically seen in alcoholics characterised by the triad of:
   1. Acute confusion
   2. Ataxia
   3. Opthalmoplegia

Wernicke encephalopathy when memory loss (global amnesia) and contabulation.

MRI shows on T2 symmetrical increased T2 signal intensity in the mammillary bodies, medial thalami tactal plate, periaqueductal area.

112. a. False b. False c. True   d. True   e. True

Dermoid/Epidermoid Cyst of Skull

Benign, slow growing, painless subcutaneous swelling, intradiploic tend to be midline in the frontotemporal location.

On CT, hypodense and non-enhancing.

On MRI, low intensity on T1 and high on T2.

113. a. False   b. True   c. True   d. True   e. True

Choroid plexus xanthogranuloma mostly found in the lateral ventricles, too small to cause any symptom. May obstructions of the foremen of monro. Spillage of debris into the cerebral spinal fluid.

114. a. False   b. True   c. False   d. True   e. False

115. a. True   b. True   c. True   d. True   e. False

Hypertensive encephalopathy (Posterior reversible encephalopathy syndrome).

Also known as hypertensive microangiopathy that results in the basal ganglin pons and cerebellum.

116. a. True   b. True   c. True   d. False   e. True

117. a. True   b. True   c. True   d. True   e. False

118. a. True   b. False   c. True   d. True   e. True

119. a. False   b. True   c. True   d. True   e. True

A pert syndrome is predomanently characterized by skull and limb malformation.associated with CNS anomalies,congenital, genitourinary anomalies, facial hypoplasia, hypertelorism, exopthalamos, croniostenosis.

120. a. True   b. True   c. True   d. False   e. False

121. a. True   b. False   c. False   d. True   e. True

122. a. False   b. True   c. True   d. True   e. True

123. a. True b. True   c. True   d. False e. True

124. a. True   b. True   c. False d. True   e. True

Also in prenatal infection, e.g., toxoplasmosis rubella, cytomegalic inclusion disease, herpes syphilis. Down syndrome, Fahr's syndrome (ferrocalcinosis), Fanconi syndrome, incontinentia pigmenti cerebral atrophy.

125. a. True   b. True   c. False d. True   e. True

Also seen in Paget's disease, lymphangioma of the tongue. Facial hemihypertrophy (unilateral prognathism), cerebral gigantism, Wiedemann-Backwith syndrome, and normal variant, etc.

126. a. True   b. True   c. False d. True   e. True

Also seen in cataract, foreign body varices, haemangioma, aneurysm atherosclerosis, collagen disease, hyperparathyroidism, metastases, multiple myeloma, milk-alkali syndrome, infections, e.g., TB abscess, neurofibroma, mucocele invading orbit. Retiroblastoma, trauma, etc.

127. a. True   b. True   c. False d. False e. True

Also seen in neurofibromatosis osteitis, thalassemia, Paget's disease, osteopetrosis, microphthalmos, radiation therapy, enucleation in childhood. While there is enlargement in thyroid—eye disease and pseudotumour.

128. a. True   b. True   c. True   d. False e. False

Also seen in amyloidosis, cretinism Down syndrome, glycogen storage disease, mucopolysaccaridosis muscular dystrophy, neoplasm, trauma, Beckwith-Wiedemann visceromegaly syndrome, etc.

129. a. True   b. True   c. False d. True   e. True

Also seen in neurofibromatosis, pseudotumour, dermoid cyst, haemangioma, etc.

130. a. False   b. True   c. True   d. True   e. True

Also seen in mumps, stone in the duct, stricture of the duct cirrhosis, nutritional deficiency, Kwashiorkor, hormonal disturbance, e.g., hypothyroidism, pregnancy sarcoidosis, alcoholism, tumour, e.g., mixed tumour, infections, e.g., suppurative Sialectasis, etc.

131. a. True   b. False   c. False   d. False   e. False

Reversal sign is seen on CT scan images and represents a diffuse decrease in density of the cerebral hemisphere with loss of grey-white differentiation and relative increase in density of the thalami, brainstem, and cerebellum. It is seen in several injury, brain asphyxia drowning, status epilepticus, bacterial meningitis, and encephalitis. It represents anoxic ischemic cerebral injury. It indicates irreversible brain damage and carries a poor prognosis.

Pancake sign is a congenital malformation of the brain, abnormal brain in a lobar holoprosencephaly associated with midline facial abnormalities. Lemon sign represents the loss of the normal convex contour of the frontal bones, with flattening or inward scalloping, associated with spina bifida and other. Hyperdense MCA sign refer to the hyperdense middle cerebral artery seen on unenhanced CT scan images in acute stroke. Medusa head sign is seen in a developmental venous anomaly where multiple tributaries arranged in a radial fashion drain into a larger vein, this sign is best on gadolinium-enhanced T1W images. Hot nose sign represents increase perfusion in the nasopharyngeal region on radionuclide scans.

132. a. True   b. True   c. True   d. True   e. False

133. a. True   b. True   c. True   d. False   e. True

134. a. False   b. False   c. False   d. True   e. True

135. a. False   b. True   c. False   d. False   e. True

Routine ultrasound scan for the diagnosis of congenital anomalies is done in second trimester. Acrania is a condition in which the flat bones of the cranial vault are partially or completely absent. Exencephaly is an early stage of anencephaly in which that the brain is located outside the skull.

136. a. True   b. False c. True   d. True   e. True

137. a. True   b. True   c. True   d. False e. True

138. a. True   b. True   c. True   d. True   e. False

139. a. True   b. False c. True   d. True   e. True

140. a. True b. True c. False d. True e. True

141. a. True   b. True   c. True   d. True   e. False

142. a. True   b. True   c. True   d. True   e. False

143. a. False b. False c. True   d. True   e. False

144. a. True   b. True   c. False d. False e. False

Tram-Track sign is composed of two enhancing areas of tumour separated from each other by the negative defect of the optic nerve. It is seen on contrast enhanced CT and MRI images. The Tram-Track sign is not specific for meningiomas and has also been described in orbital pseudotumour, perioptic neuritis sarcoidosis, leukaemia, metastasis, lymphoma, and perioptic haemorrhages.

145. a. True   b. True   c. False d. True   e. False

146. a. True   b. True   c. True   d. False e. False

147. a. False b. False c. False d. True   e. True

148. a. True   b. True   c. True   d. False e. True

149. a. True   b. True   c. True   d. False e. True

150. a. True   b. True   c. True   d. False e. True

Neuroendocrine tumours (NET) are very rare and arise usually in the gastrointestinal and respiratory tracts. Tumours with neuroendocrine differentiation frequently express chromogranin A (CgA), synaptophysin. These tumours show frequent incidence of metastasis in the liver.

151. a. True   b. False   c. True   d. True   e. True

152. a. True   b. True   c. False   d. False   e. True

Also seen in chronic sclerosing osteomyelitis, e.g., brucella, TB typhoid.

Seen also in sarcoidosis sickle cell anaemia, renal osteodystrophy, osteopetrosis, fluorosis, myelosclerosis, etc.

153. a. False   b. False   c. True   d. True   e. True

154. a. False   b. False   c. True   d. True   e. True

Also seen in syringomyelia, hydromyelia, dwarfism, neurofibromatosis. Tumour of the spinal canal, e.g., dermoid, lipoma, meningioma.

155. a. True   b. True   c. True   d. False   e. False

156. a. True   b. False   c. True   d. True   e. False

157. a. True   b. True   c. True   d. False   e. False

Rugger-jersey spine is sclerotic superior and inferior end plates of vertebrae. Rat-tail signs is irregularly marginated tapering ends.

Rigler's sign is visualisation of both sides of bowel wall on CT and radiography in presence of a pneumoperitonium.

Rice grain calcification in the soft tissue usually in the calf region usually seen in worm infestation, e.g., cysticercosis.

Reverse 3 sign appearance of inner margin of duodenal loop from enlarged head of pancreas with tethering at ampulla.

158. a. True   b. True   c. True   d. True   e. False

Berry aneurysm is an intracranial in location within the circle of wills usually particularly at the junction of major vessels in the anterior circulation. May be associated with co-arctation of aorta. Blade of glass sign seen in active Paget's disease of bone usually seen in diaphysis is wedge shaped.

Anteater nose sign seen on the lateral view of foot, elongated anterior, superior process of calcaneus seen in tarsal coalition.

159. a. True   b. True   c. False   d. False   e. False

McCune-Albright syndrome consists of at least two of the following three features:
1. Polyostatic fibrous dysplasia.
2. Café-au-lait skin pigmentation.
3. Autonomous endocrine hyperfunction (e.g., gonadotropin-independent precocious puberty).

Fibrous dysplasia is a disease of bone in which normal bone is replaced by abnormal fibrous tissue. The disease may be monostotic or polyostotic. There can be 3 radiographic patterns: sclerotic, cystic, and pagetoid.

On CT scan, it has typically 'ground-glass appearance'.

160. a. True   b. True   c. False   d. False   e. True

Also associated with polydactyly hydromyelia, macroglossia, localised gigantism, Leontiasis ossea.

On MRI shows mass lesion in one side of the cerebellum usually.

Linear striations resembling 'tiger stripes' with isotense bands with area of hyperintense bands with area of hyperintensity on T2W+ image corresponding to hypointensity on T1W+ image. No enhancement following injection of contrast. No edema revealed around the lesion should be differentiated from medulloblastoma, Astrocytoma, cerebritis, Ependymoma, etc.

161. a. True   b. True   c. False   d. True   e. True

162. a. False   b. False   c. False   d. True   e. True

163. a. True   b. True   c. True   d. False   e. False

164. a. True   b. False   c. True   d. True   e. True

165. a. True   b. True   c. True   d. False   e. True

166.	a. True	b. True	c. False	d. True	e. True
167.	a. True	b. True	c. True	d. True	e. False
168.	a. False	b. False	c. False	d. True	e. True
169.	a. True	b. True	c. True	d. True	e. False
170.	a. True	b. True	c. True	d. False	e. True
171.	a. True	b. True	c. False	d. True	e. False

Also seen in neurofibromatosis, Dandy-Walker syndrome, premature craniocytosis. Hydrocephalus, Paget's disease (Tam-o-Shanter skull). A fibrous dysplasia (Leontiasis ossea). Achondroplasia, associated with causes of hemiatrophy or hemihypertrophy of the cerebral hemisphere including Struge-Weber syndrome. Also in cerebral palsy, etc.

172.	a. True	b. True	c. False	d. True	e. True
173.	a. True	b. False	c. True	d. True	e. True
174.	a. True	b. True	c. True	d. False	e. True
175.	a. True	b. True	c. False	d. True	e. True

Also in fibrous dysplasia, cholesteatoma, depressed fracture, growing fracture. Archnoid cyst, Brown tumour, osteomyelitis including TB tumours including metastasis, plasmocytoma, etc.

176.	a. True	b. True	c. False	d. True	e. True

In cysticercosis only is calcified. Dracunculus medinesis (guina worm) madina worm is not a parasite and calcified in the soft tissue give an elongated strip of calcium density.

177.	a. False	b. True	c. False	d. True	e. False
178.	a. True	b. True	c. True	d. True	e. False
179.	a. True	b. False	c. True	d. True	e. False

Is primary benign tumour, are located at the foramen of monro in 99% of cases.

The majority of cases are found incidentally and are asymptomatic. Their position in the roof of the third ventricle. Can on occasion result in sudden obstructive hydrocephalus. The headaches tend to be positional.

180. a. True   b. False   c. True   d. True   e. True

181. a. True   b. True   c. True   d. False   e. True

Is a condition in which a subarachnoid recess extends into the sella and compresses the pituitary. There is usually enlargement of the fossa, which can be stimulate expansion by a tumour.

The normal maximum length of the sella in a true sagittal plain is about 17 mm and the depth 14 mm.

There is no erosion of the lamina dura and no posterior displacement of the dorsum sellae.

On MRI demonstrate the sella to be filled with CSF and the infundibulum can be seen to traverse the space. And this is known as the infundibulum sign.

182. a. True   b. True   c. True   d. True   e. False

183. a. True   b. True   c. True   d. False   e. False

184. a. True   b. True   c. False   d. True   e. False

185. a. True   b. True   c. False   d. True   e. True

186. a. True   b. True   c. True   d. True   e. False

Cord sign refers to cord-like hyperattenuation within a dural venous sinus on non-contrast enhanced CT due to dural venous thrombosis.

187. a. True   b. False   c. True   d. False   e. True

Radicular cyst is odontogenic lesion as well as ameloblastoma. The rest are non-odontogenic lesions as in fibrous dysplasia (cherubism), mandibular metastasis, periapical abscess, giant cell granuloma, squamous cell carcinoma invading mandible, traumatic bone cyst, etc.

188. a. True   b. True   c. False   d. True   e. False

189. a. True   b. False   c. True   d. False   e. False

Is lytic benign lesion of the jaw, it does not contain any fluid and result from remodelling of the bone by adjacent salivary gland tissue. Frequently seen in middle-aged men.

190. a. True   b. True   c. False   d. True   e. True

191. a. True   b. True   c. True   d. True   e. False

192. a. False   b. True   c. True   d. False   e. True

193. a. False   b. False   c. True   d. True   e. True

194. a. True   b. False   c. True   d. True   e. True

195. a. True   b. True   c. False   d. True   e. True

196. a. False   b. False   c. False   d. True   e. False

197. a. False   b. True   c. True   d. True   e. True

198. a. False   b. False   c. False   d. True   e. True

199. a. True   b. True   c. True   d. False   e. True

200. a. False   b. False   c. True   d. False   e. False

201. a. False   b. True   c. False   d. False   e. True

202. a. False   b. True   c. True   d. True   e. True

203. a. True   b. False   c. False   d. False   e. True

204. a. True   b. True   c. True   d. True   e. False

205. a. True   b. True   c. False   d. True   e. True

206. a. False   b. True   c. True   d. True   e. False

207. a. True   b. True   c. False   d. True   e. True

208. a. False   b. True   c. False   d. False   e. True

209. a. True   b. True   c. True   d. False   e. True

210. a. True   b. True   c. False   d. True   e. True

211. a. True   b. False   c. False   d. False   e. False

212. a. True   b. False   c. False   d. True   e. False

213. a. False   b. False   c. False   d. True   e. False

214. a. True   b. True   c. False   d. True   e. True

215. a. False   b. True   c. False   d. True   e. False

216. a. True   b. True   c. False   d. True   e. True

217. a. False   b. True   c. False   d. True   e. True

218. a. True   b. True   c. True   d. False   e. True

Most probably due to an immune-mediated endotheliopathy that involves the microvessels of the brain, retina, and inner ear.

Symptoms include memory impairment, confusion, behavioural disturbances, ataxia, dysarthria, and psychosis.

Multiple sclerosis (MS) is the most important differential diagnosis.

219. a. False   b. False   c. True   d. True   e. True

1. In anterior hip dislocation:
   a) Diagnosed confidently by conventional radiography.
   b) Posterior hip dislocation are much more common than anterior.
   c) CT provide an accurate means of evaluating the associated fractures.
   d) Avascular necrosis of femoral head is recognised complication.
   e) Associated with spina bifida oculta.

2. Dislocation of the bone is a feature of following fracture:
   a) Bennett's.
   b) Galeazzi.
   c) Smith's.
   d) Colles.
   e) Barton's.

3. In rickets:
   a) Swelling of the wrists and ankles.
   b) Periosteal reaction is a feature.
   c) Increase the distance between the end of shaft and epiphyseal centre.
   d) Early dentition.
   e) Seen in anticonvulsant drug therapy.

4. In protrusion acetabuli the following are true:
   a) Can be unilateral.
   b) Seen in collagen disease.
   c) May be asymptomatic.
   d) Avascular necrosis is a common cause.
   e) Seen in Marfan's syndrome.

5. The following are true in erosive osteoarthritis:
   a) Commonly occurs in men over the age of 60.
   b) Usually involve the hip joints.
   c) Typically bilateral.
   d) Marginal erosion of the bones is common.
   e) Typically rheumatoid factor negative.

6. In Diffuse Idiopathic Skeletal Hyperostosis (DISH), the following are true:
   a) Associated with acromegaly.
   b) Associated with ankylosing spondylitis.
   c) Associate with rheumatoid arthritis.
   d) Thick skull vault due to hyperostosis frontalis interna.
   e) Common in old Caucasian males.

7. In osteochondritis dissecans:
   a) In the elbow, the trochlea is the most common site.
   b) The hip is the most commonly involve joint.
   c) In the knee, the medial femoral condyle is the most common position.
   d) In the ankle, the talus is most usually involved site.
   e) Commonly affected male over 50 years.

8. Pseudofracture (Looser's zone) are seen in:
   a) Albright's syndrome.
   b) Spondylosis.
   c) Osteomalacia.
   d) Sudeck's atrophy.
   e) Rickets.

9. In Caisson's disease:
   a) Lesions more common in femur than humerus.
   b) Sclerotic areas in epiphysis is a common feature.
   c) Usually symmetrical.
   d) May give rise to osteolytic areas in medullary cavities.
   e) Give rise to fragmented epiphyses in children.

10. Wormian bones are seen in:
    a) Rickets.
    b) Osteogenesis imperfecta.
    c) Cretinism.

d) Aqueduct stenosis.
   e) Cleidocranial dysostosis.

11. Bilateral thickening of the heel pad (greater than 2.2 cm) seen in:
    a) Thyroid acropachy.
    b) Acromegaly.
    c) Turner's syndrome.
    d) Dilantin therapy.
    e) Mycetoma.

12. In hypertrophic osteoarthropathy:
    a) Clubbing finger.
    b) Lamellar periosteal proliferation of new bone.
    c) Sparing the mandible.
    d) Is painless swelling of the limbs.
    e) Bone scan shows decrease periarticular uptake.

13. Condition involves skin and bone:
    a) Mastocytosis.
    b) Fibrous dysplasia.
    c) Actiromycosis.
    d) Leprosy.
    e) Plasmocytoma.

14. Bone within a bone appearance seen:
    a) Ankylosing apondylitis.
    b) Normal neonate.
    c) Cleidocranial dystosis.
    d) Sickle cell anaemia.
    e) Osteoporosis.

15. In nail-patella syndrome (Fong's disease) called (Hood syndrome) or elbow-patella syndrome:
    a) Bilateral iliac horns.
    b) Abnormal gait.
    c) Abnormal pigmentation of iris.
    d) Long 5th metacarpal.
    e) Evident in the 1st year of life.

16. The following may give rise to fractures:
    a) Lead poisoning.
    b) Anticonvulsant therapy.
    c) Hypophosphatasia.
    d) Osteoporosis.
    e) Renal disease.

17. In volar plate fracture:
    a) Small fragment of bone is avulsed from palmar aspect of base of middle finger.
    b) Is hyperextension injury.
    c) Joint stability is a common complication.
    d) Is a stress fracture.
    e) Also called Bennett's fracture.

18. In pachydermoperiostosis:
    a) Associated with congenital heart disease.
    b) Associated with congenital hip dislocation.
    c) Causing severe pain with swelling.
    d) Sparing the epiphysis and ligament innervations.
    e) Clubbing fingers.

19. Solitary sclerotic bone lesion with a lucent centre seen in:
    a) Osteoid osteoma.
    b) Osteoblastoma.
    c) Myeloma.
    d) Brodie's abscess.
    e) Caries sicca.

20. In hyperparathyroidism:
    a) The tertiary condition may result from renal failure.
    b) There is often a family history.
    c) When primary usually due to an adenoma.
    d) May be associated with islet cell tumour.
    e) May be associated with peptic ulcer.

21. Caffey's disease is associated with:
    a) Raised ESR.
    b) Pleural effusion is common.
    c) Only in enchondral bone.

d) Usually occurs after 6 months of age.
e) Due to concealed trauma.

22. The following favour a diagnosis of psoriasis rather than rheumatoid:
    a) Skin nodules.
    b) Sacroilitis.
    c) Involvement of distal interphalangeal (DIP) joints.
    d) Symmetrical joint disease.
    e) Calcaneal spur.

23. The following are true:
    a) The commonest site of giant cell tumour in the spine.
    b) Aneurysmal bone cyst arises most commonly in the vertebral body.
    c) Osteoid osteoma of the spine occurs most commonly in the neural arch.
    d) Chondroblastoma arises usually in metaphysis.
    e) Fibrous cortical defects arise usually in the diaphysis of the long bones.

24. Generalised increase bony density in children seen in:
    a) Lead poisoning.
    b) Cretinism.
    c) Paget's
    d) Treated rickets.
    e) Hypervitaminosis D.

25. The following may give rise to osteosclerosis:
    a) Myelosclerosis.
    b) Engelmann's disease.
    c) Mastocytosis.
    d) Vitamin C deficiency.
    e) Turner's disease.

26. The following cause periosteal reaction:
    a) Hodgkin's disease.
    b) Yaws.
    c) Bronchogenic carcinoma.
    d) Psoriasis.
    e) Primary hypothyroidism.

27. The following features favour myeloma rather than metastases:
    a) Jaw involvement.
    b) Vertebral pedicle involvement.
    c) Raised alkaline phosphatase.
    d) Diffuse osteoporosis.
    e) Soft tissue swelling.

28. The following are features of haemophilic arthropathy of the knee:
    a) Articular cartilage calcification.
    b) Coarse trabeculation of epiphysis.
    c) Increase in size of epiphysis.
    d) Shallow intercondylar notch.
    e) Growth lines in the metaphysis.

29. Multiple osteosclerotic bone lesion seen in:
    a) Brown tumour.
    b) Osteoblastoma.
    c) Plasmacytoma.
    d) Mastocytosis.
    e) Chondromyxoid fibroma.

30. In sacroiliac joints disease:
    a) Whipple's disease
    b) Reiter's syndrome
    c) Ulcerative colitis.
    d) Paraplagia.
    e) Hypoparathyroidism.

31. 31.In sacroiliac joint disease:
    a) Ankylosing spondylitis.
    b) Psoriasis.
    c) Gout.
    d) Crohn's disease.
    e) Benign prostatic hypertrophy.

32. In hemihypertrophy;
    a) Wilm's tumour.
    b) Hypospadias.
    c) Pituitary adenoma.
    d) Medullary sponge kidney.
    e) Hepatoblastoma.

33. In the shoulder the following are true:
    a) Labral tears can occur in the absence of shoulder instability.
    b) A Bankart lesion is a tear or separation of the posterior inferior glenoid labram.
    c) The superior glenohumeral ligament (GHL) and middle GHL may be absent in normal individuals.
    d) SLAP tears are tears of the biceps labral complex and often occur after a forced extension injury.
    e) CT arthrography is less sensitive than plain MRI at detecting labral tears.

34. Morquio-Brailsford disease the following are true:
    a) Platyspondyly.
    b) Epiphyseal fragmentation.
    c) Thin narrow limb bones.
    d) Normal lumbar spine.
    e) Normal hand x-ray.

35. A 3-week-old baby shows periosteal reaction along the femur this may be:
    a) A normal variant.
    b) Hypervitaminosis A.
    c) Hypervitaminous D.
    d) Scurvy.
    e) Leukaemia.

36. Features of homocystinuria are:
    a) Dwarfism.
    b) Pectus excavatum.
    c) Ectopia lentis.
    d) Kyphoscoliosis.
    e) Increase in bone density.

37. The following are features of Hurler's syndrome:
    a) Normally appears at the age of 10–15 years.
    b) Coxa vara.
    c) Spatulate rib configuration.
    d) J-shaped sella.
    e) Trident hand.

38. In haemophilia:
    a) Changes most frequent in shoulders.
    b) Enlarged nutrient foramen occurs.
    c) Delayed epiphyseal fusion occurs.
    d) Periaticular erosion occurs.
    e) Pseudotumours are common.

39. Increase in the size of a limb may occur:
    a) Neuroblastomatosis.
    b) Osteopetrosis.
    c) Lymphangioma.
    d) Lipomatosis.
    e) Flourosis.

40. The following are associated with osteomalacia:
    a) Hemochromatosis.
    b) Jejunal diverticulosis.
    c) Neurofibromatosis.
    d) Acute renal failure.
    e) Anticonvulsant therapy.

41. Persistence of congenital dislocation of hip may be associated with:
    a) The presence of a limbus vertebra.
    b) Bowing femur.
    c) Kyhoscoliosis.
    d) Coxa vara.
    e) Osteopenia.

42. In children decreased density of the metaphyses may be seen in:
    a) Neurofibromatosis.
    b) Acute leukaemia.
    c) Syphilis
    d) Amyloid disease.
    e) Rickets.

43. Precocious puberty may be seen in:
    a) Sturge-Weber syndrome.
    b) Renal Osteodystrophy.
    c) A large calcified pineal gland.
    d) With calcification in the base of the brain.
    e) Fibrous dysplasia.

44. The following are true in relation to diastrophic dwarfism:
    a) Flat foot.
    b) Hitch-hiker's thumb.
    c) Cauliflower ear.
    d) Squaring shape vertebra with scoliosis.
    e) Madelung's deformities.

45. In myositis ossificance progressiva (fibrodysplasia ossificans progressiva) the following are true:
    a) Short hallux is common.
    b) Not involved the larynx or the tongue.
    c) Characterised by painless swelling without tenderness in the shoulders and the thorax with occasional pyrexia.
    d) The diaphragm is not affected.
    e) Short thumb is association.

46. Signs of Perthe's disease are:
    a) Gage sign (defect in lateral part of the epiphysis V shape).
    b) Caffey's sign (crescent sign).
    c) Usually bilateral.
    d) Metaphyseal cysts.
    e) Bony scan is highly sensitive.

47. Cone-shaped epiphysis seen in:
    a) Achondroplasia.
    b) Osteopetrosis.
    c) Down syndrome.
    d) Dactylitis.
    e) Hypervitaminosis.

48. Charcot joint occur in:
    a) Syringomyelia.
    b) Leprosy.
    c) Acromegaly.
    d) Poliomylitis.
    e) Tabes dorsalis.

49. Blow out lesion of bone seen in:
    a) Giant cell tumour.
    b) Plasmocytoma.
    c) Hydatid cyst.

d) Osteoid osteoma.
e) Ossifying fibroma.

50. Symmetrical expansion of the lower femora occurs in:
    a) Gaucher's disease.
    b) Diaphyseal aclasia.
    c) Pyles disease.
    d) Leukaemia.
    e) Syphilis.

51. The following are true of an aneurysmal bone cyst:
    a) Is usually situated in the diaphysis.
    b) Is multi centric.
    c) Is caused by aneurysmal dilatation of a nutrient artery.
    d) A common benign tumour of vertebral body.
    e) Is more likely to be found in a girl of 15 than a man of 55.

52. The following may occur in Turner's syndrome:
    a) Horseshoe kidney.
    b) Hypertelorism.
    c) Thin ribs.
    d) Shortening of 4th metacarpal.
    e) Early fusion of epiphysis.

53. In alkaptonuria (Ochronosis):
    a) Severe narrowing of intervertebral disk space.
    b) Hypertrophic changes in humeral head.
    c) Generalised increase bony density.
    d) Multiple vacuum phenomena are common.
    e) Is due to renal failure.

54. The following condition more likely to terminate in leukaemia:
    a) Osteopetrosis.
    b) Mast Cell Reticulosis.
    c) Myelosclerosis.
    d) Mongolism.
    e) Marfan's disease.

55. Congenital dislocation of the hip joint occurs in:
    a) Arthrogryposis.
    b) Perthe's disease.

c) Fanconi syndrome of congenital Aplastic anaemia.
d) Marfan's syndrome.
e) Cerebral palsy.

56. The following are true in Morquio syndrome:
    a) The onset usually between 2 and 4 years.
    b) Keratan Sulphate is present in the urine.
    c) The dwarfing is due to platyspondyly.
    d) Normal Intelligence.
    e) Associated with bilateral congenital dislocation of the hip.

57. Joints laxity occurs in:
    a) Morquio syndrome.
    b) Marfan's syndrome.
    c) Homocystine Urea.
    d) Hemophilia.
    e) Ehlar-Donler syndrome.

58. In diffuse idiopathic skeletal hyperostosis (DISH):
    a) May be due to altered vitamin A metabolism.
    b) Commonly in children.
    c) Big heel spurs.
    d) Spur on anterior surface of patella.
    e) Whiskering at iliac crest (fringing deformity).

59. Calcified lymph glands occur in:
    a) Histoplasmosis.
    b) Filariasis.
    c) Thyroid metasis.
    d) Multiple myeloma.
    e) Sarcoidosis.

60. Localised elongation of bone occur in:
    a) Macrodystrophia lipomatosa.
    b) Neurofibromatosis.
    c) Still's disease.
    d) Marfan's disease.
    e) Albright syndrome.

61. The following are true in dysplasia epiphysis hemimelica (Trevor disease):
    a) Shortening of the affected bone.
    b) Histoligically indistinguishable from osteochondroma.
    c) Limited joint mobility.
    d) The arm is the most commonly affected.
    e) When it is multiple usually symmetrical.

62. Retardation of bone age commonly occurs in:
    a) Malnutrition.
    b) Treatment of steroids.
    c) Perthe's disease.
    d) Chromophobe adenoma.
    e) Albright's fibrous dysplasia syndrome.

63. Turner's syndrome includes:
    a) Short metacarpals.
    b) Madelung deformity.
    c) Coartation of aorta.
    d) Hypotelorism.
    e) Pes cavus (club foot).

64. Carpal fusion occurs in:
    a) Turner's syndrome.
    b) Still's disease.
    c) Psoriasis.
    d) Arthrogryposis.
    e) Ellis-van Creveld syndrome (Chondroectodermal dysplasia).

65. Homocystinuria is typically associated with:
    a) Protrusio acetabuli.
    b) Osteoporosis.
    c) Premature vascular calcifications.
    d) Arachnodactyly.
    e) Flat foots.

66. There is an association between Marfan's and:
    a) Short patellar ligament.
    b) Aneurysm of the ascending aorta.
    c) Dextrocardia.

d) Pes excavation.
e) Kyphoscoliosis.

67. Extreme joint mobility may be present in:
    a) Ehlers-Danlos syndrome.
    b) Gargoylism.
    c) Marfan's syndrome.
    d) Homocystinuria.
    e) Nail-patella syndrome (Fong disease).

68. Change in the metaphyses are commonly seen in:
    a) Histocytosis X.
    b) Hypophosphatia.
    c) Neurofibromatosis.
    d) Hyperphosphatasia.
    e) Renal osteodystrophy.

69. There is a well-recognised association between congenital dislocation of the hip and:
    a) Neurogical manifestation.
    b) Racial difference.
    c) Male preponderance.
    d) Acetabular dysplasia as the primary lesion.
    e) Breech deliveries.

70. Short clavicles are seen in:
    a) Diaphyseal aclasis (heridetary multiple exostosis).
    b) Pykenodysostosis.
    c) Cleido-cranial dysostosis.
    d) Pseudo-hypoparathyroidism.
    e) Trisomy 13–15.

71. An expanding sclerotic lesion in a rib can occur in:
    a) Hodgkin's disease.
    b) Eosinophil granuloma.
    c) Metastatic hypernephroma.
    d) Osteoid osteoma.
    e) Hyperparathyroidism.

72. In Osteochondromatosis of the knee:
    a) Usually pre-malignant.
    b) An affinity for small joints.
    c) Joint effusion is rare.
    d) Usually multiple joints affected.
    e) Mild pain, swelling, and limitation of movement are the usual presenting complaints.

73. The following cause pulmonary lesions, osseous lesions, and diabetes insipidus:
    a) Histocytosis.
    b) Sarcoid.
    c) Renal failure.
    d) Amyloid.
    e) Neurofibromatosis.

74. Signs of loosing hip arthroplastic:
    a) A zone of lucency more than 2 mm thick outlines the prosthesis strongly indicating loosing.
    b) Cement fracture.
    c) Progressive widening of lucency.
    d) Unifocal rapid and progressive resorption of bone indicating particle-related inflammatory disease (granulomatosis).
    e) CT scan is the examination of choice in identifying an infected prosthesis.

75. The following statements may be true concerning Wegner's granuloma:
    a) The lung changes usually multifocal partly air-spaces opacities.
    b) The pleural effusion is usually exudative.
    c) Otitis media is common.
    d) Renal failure is the usual cause of death in Wegner's granuloma.
    e) Migratory polyarthopathy is common.

76. In osteoid osteoma:
    a) Common above 50 years.
    b) Contains a central nidus.
    c) Produce cortical thickening.
    d) The pain is worse at night.
    e) Commonly in the spine.

77. Neuropathic joints may occur in:
    a) Poliomyelitis.
    b) Syringomyelia.
    c) Neurofibromatosis.
    d) Diabetic.
    e) Osteogenesis imperecta.

78. In haemochromatosis:
    a) 50% of patients affected the joints.
    b) Sacro iliac joints are rarely affected.
    c) Cardiac calcification may be seen.
    d) Hepatoma is common.
    e) Interpharyngeal joints are spared.

79. The following are true in gout:
    a) Chondocalcinosis.
    b) Podagra symptoms are common.
    c) Calcified deposits in gouty tophi in about 1%.
    d) Secondary to myxedema.
    e) Ischemic necrosis of femoral head.

80. In pigmented villonodular synovitis:
    a) Usually has soft tissue swelling.
    b) Give rise to clear cut bone defects.
    c) Usually occurs in young patients.
    d) Is associated with calcification.
    e) May be associated with an effusion.

81. Osteogenesis imperfecta seen:
    a) Multiple fractures sparing ribs and skull.
    b) Wormian bones are always present.
    c) Vertebral fractures are late presentation.
    d) Blue sclera, dental abnormalities, lax joints are commonly present.
    e) Death in uterus may be found.

82. In Sudeck's atrophy the following are true:
    a) Subperiosteal resorption.
    b) Joint effusion.
    c) Translucent bands in the metaphysis in an adolescent.
    d) Painful swelling of the limb.
    e) May occur after minimal trauma.

83. Solitary radiolucent metaphyseal band seen:
    a) Normal neonate.
    b) Healing rickets.
    c) Metastatic neuroblastoma.
    d) Leukaemia.
    e) Mucupolysachariodosis.

84. In progeria:
    a) Generalised bony sclerosis.
    b) Is as rare collagen disease.
    c) Associated with neurofibromatosis.
    d) Much common in male.
    e) Wormian bones.

85. The following are true in Sjoreen syndrome:
    a) Xerorhinia.
    b) Xeropthalmia.
    c) Xerostomia.
    d) Common in young male.
    e) Honeycomb lungs on CT scan.

86. The following statements are true:
    a) Lipohaemoarthrosis may be seen in the shoulder joints in the absence of an intra articular fracture.
    b) Elevation of the fat line of the radial collateral ligament is suggestive of a scaphoid fracture.
    c) The posterior oblique view of the pelvis is best to demonstrate the sacroiliac joint.
    d) On Lateral plain x-ray of elbow any posterior fat pad, regard is pathological.
    e) Mediastinal emphysema associated with diabetic coma.

87. Solitary dense metaphyseal band seen:
    a) Lead posisoning.
    b) Osteopetrosis.
    c) Hyperparathyroidism.
    d) Normal infants.
    e) Hypervitaminosis D.

88. In triplane fracture:
    a) Old male patient likely affected.
    b) Common in osteomalacia.
    c) Around the knee joint.
    d) Always need operative reduction internal fixation.
    e) Conventional radiography is the study of choice.

89. In pelvic rib (digit):
    a) An iliac horn (Fong's disease).
    b) Traumatic in origin.
    c) Bilaterally.
    d) Associated with progressive myositis ossificans.
    e) Asymptomatic.

90. The following are true in epidermal inclusion cyst:
    a) Is an expansile cystic lesion in the terminal phalanx of the index finger is the characteristic location.
    b) Associated with penetrating trauma.
    c) Pain at night typically relieved by aspirin.
    d) Impossible to be differentiated from multiple enchondroma.
    e) It can occur in the calvarium.

91. In sternomanubrial dislocation:
    a) Associated with pes cavus.
    b) Associated with rheumatoid arthritis.
    c) Lateral view of the CXR may confirm the diagnosis with certainty.
    d) May be associated with fractures of posterior aspect of the ribs and pleural effusion.
    e) Always treated by closed reduction.

92. The following are true in necrotizing fasciitis:
    a) In children associated with necrotizing enterocolitis.
    b) Tuberculosis is most common association.
    c) Severe localise pain is always present.
    d) Pulmonary septic emboli is a complication.
    e) Non-enhanced CT scan is the study of choice.

93. Giant bone island the following are true:
    a) Painful at night.
    b) Commonly in skull vault.

c) Response to treatment by cortisone.
d) Radionuclide bone scan usually shows no increased uptake.
e) Periosteal reaction locally.

94. In melorheostosis:
    a) Common in black over 50 years.
    b) Common in lower limbs.
    c) Associated with muscle contractures.
    d) Scoliosis.
    e) Bone scan is negative.

95. The following are true in fibrous dysplasia:
    a) Premalignant.
    b) Solitary usually.
    c) Commonly involve the pelvis and femora.
    d) Associated with skin pigmentation.
    e) Associated with neurofibromatosis.

96. In ankylosing spondylitis:
    a) Mostly young male Caucasians.
    b) HLA-B 27 positive in > 90%.
    c) Bamboo spine on AP view.
    d) Erosions of the temperomandibular joints.
    e) Vertebra planna.

97. Rheumatoid arthritis may present with:
    a) Myopathy.
    b) Encephalitis.
    c) Sudden pain in calf.
    d) Large pericardial effusion.
    e) Hypochromic anaemia.

98. The following may have soft tissue calcification in the hands (about the fingertips):
    a) Ochinonosis.
    b) Hypoparathyroidism.
    c) Raynauds phenomenon.
    d) Chronic renal failure.
    e) Primary hyperparathyroidism.

99. The following vascular calcifications are associated with present of phleboliths:
    a) Frostbite.
    b) Gout.
    c) Hypervitaminosis D.
    d) Maffucci's syndrome.
    e) Buerger's disease.

100. The following are true in anterior shoulder dislocation:
    a) Old males commonly affected.
    b) Associated with Hill-Sachs defect is common.
    c) Associated with rheumatoid arthritis.
    d) Bilateral 10%.
    e) Associated with Bankart lesion.

101. The following are true in carpal tunnel syndrome:
    a) Obesity common associated condition.
    b) Seen in associated with hypothyroidism.
    c) Common in diabetic patient.
    d) Not response to conservative measures.
    e) Leukaemia is a recognised causes.

102. In achondroplasia:
    a) Recurrent otitis media.
    b) Short stature.
    c) Frontal bossing.
    d) Long phalanges.
    e) Wide interpediculate distance.

103. In non-union fracture the following are true:
    a) In the skull called growing fracture.
    b) Cigarette smoking place patient at high risk.
    c) Infection is common associated cause.
    d) MRI is best modality for diagnosis.
    e) Underlying pathology is always present.

104. Bilateral coxa vara seen in:
    a) Hypothyroidism.
    b) Hyperphosphatasia.
    c) Hyperparathyroidism.

d) Achondroplasia.
   e) Trevor's disease (dysplasia epiphyseal is hemimelica).

105. In pigmented villonodular synovitis:
   a) Non-articular pain and swelling around a major joint usually the knee or hip.
   b) Plain radiograph shows scalloped erosions on both side of joints associated with soft tissue swelling.
   c) In the earliest cases the narrowed joint space and the erosion of articular margins are seen on plain radiograph.
   d) Calcification within the hypertrophic soft tissues is common.
   e) Associated with Stills disease.

106. In diaphyseal aclasia:
   a) Family history.
   b) Premalignant.
   c) Hypermobility of the joints.
   d) Sparing of the spine.
   e) Exostosis point away from the joint.

107. In cysticerosis:
   a) The larval form of taenia solium by ingestion of infested pork that has been incompletely cooked.
   b) Meningoencephalitis can occur.
   c) Diffusely scattered 'riselike' calcifications in the muscles.
   d) Can be differentiated from Loa Loa infestation on plain radiograph.
   e) Adult worm residue in the liver.

108. In chance fracture of lumbar vertebra:
   a) Abrupt deceleration against an automobile seat belt.
   b) Commonly involve any vertebra from T12-L4.
   c) A good lateral view generally is diagnostic.
   d) Asymmetry of the psoas muscle thickness and density.
   e) Neurological deficient is usually present.

109. Tarsal coalitions are true.
   a) Most are asymptomatic.
   b) Pes cavus is common.
   c) Associated with fibrous dysplasia.

d) Plain radiograph, the talar beak on dorsum of talus indicating the tarsal coalition is likely present.
e) Bilateral is common.

110. The following are true in Ewing's Sarcoma:
a) Commonly involves metaphysis of long bones in children.
b) Any bone can involve sparing the mandible.
c) Metastases is common at the time of diagnosis.
d) Low signal intensity on T1WI and heterogeneous gadolinium enhancement.
e) Lamellated or sunburst periosteal reaction on plain radiograph is common.

111. In lipohemarthrosis:
a) Presence of fat and fluid in the joint capsule following trauma.
b) Always indicating fracture.
c) Fat/fluid level can be seen on plain radiograph.
d) MRI have been used to diagnose the underlying occult fracture.
e) CT scan to indentify occult fractures.

112. In cleidocranial dysostosis the following are true:
a) Osteoporosis.
b) Short clavicles.
c) Iliac horns.
d) Coxa valga deformity.
e) Fused symphysis pubic joint.

113. In complex regional pain syndrome (Sudeck's atrophy):
a) Osteopenia.
b) Causalgia.
c) Located proximal to the fracture.
d) Positive bony scan.
e) Can be diagnosed by conventional radiographs.

114. Following signs may be associated in ankylosing spondylitis:
a) Bamboo spine.
b) Trolley-track sign.
c) Shiny-corner sign.
d) Both sacroiliac joints are always symmetrically involve.
e) Periosteal whiskering sign.

115. A 10-year-old mentally retarded girl with severe pain in the left knee joint. The x-ray of the knee shows localised osteoporosis and no bony injury. All the biochemical tests are negative. The following may be a possible cause:
    a) Transient osteoporosis.
    b) Disuse osteoporosis due to underlying osteochondritis.
    c) Tear of cruciate or menisci.
    d) Sudeck's strophy.
    e) Whipple's disease.

116. The following statements are true regarding Gaucher's disease:
    a) Young Jewish females are peculiarly susceptible to this hereditary condition.
    b) Vertebra plana.
    c) Pathological fractures.
    d) Acro-osteolysis.
    e) Flask-shaped femora.

117. Separation of symphysis pubis on a child may be seen in:
    a) Cleidocranial dystosis.
    b) Physiological.
    c) Epispadias.
    d) Exstrophy of the bladder.
    e) Ostitis pubis.

118. The following statements are true of fibrous dysplasia:
    a) Most skeletal lesions become apparent childhood.
    b) Hyperstosis of the base of the skull may be seen in infancy.
    c) Sexual precocity (Albright syndrome) is more common in males than females.
    d) The epiphysis is spared in childhood.
    e) Calcification within the lesion is an uncommon feature.

119. In unicameral bone cyst (simple bone cyst):
    a) Is a common primary bone tumour affected male more than female between 5 and 10 years.
    b) Malignant transformation can occur.
    c) When it is multiple the humerus is always involved.
    d) Metaphyseal in location away from the epiphyseal plate.
    e) It is also called brown tumour.

120. In calcium Hydroxyapatite Deposition Disease (HADD):
    a) Also known as tumoural calcinosis.
    b) Also known as Heterotopic ossification trabeculation.
    c) Usually self limiting condition.
    d) The knee is the most common site.
    e) Associated with collagen vascular disease.

121. Extra intestinal manifestations of ulcerative colitis:
    a) Migratory arthritis.
    b) Sacroilitis and ankylosing spondylitis.
    c) Peptic ulcer.
    d) Uveitis.
    e) Sclerosing cholangitis.

122. In gamekeeper's thumb / Skier's thumb (Break-dancer's thumb):
    a) Chronic injury to ulnar collateral ligament of thumb.
    b) May be seen in rheumatoid arthritis.
    c) May comprise up to 50% of injuries to hand in skiers.
    d) Associated with Bennett's fracture dislocation.
    e) Seen also in pseudo-gout.

123. Loss of axillary hair occurs in:
    a) Addison's disease.
    b) Cushing's syndrome.
    c) Hypopituitarism.
    d) Turner's syndrome.
    e) Polycystic ovaries.

124. Chondrocalcinosis seen in:
    a) Hypertrophic asteoarthropathy.
    b) Gout.
    c) Wilson's disease.
    d) Primary hyperparathyroidism.
    e) Haemochromatosis.

125. In pseudogout (articular chondrocalcinosis / idiopathic chondrocalcinosis):
    a) Associated with presence of calcium pyrophosphate crystals.
    b) Associated mostly with osteoarthritis.
    c) Sparing the shoulder joint.
    d) Can involve the annulus of the intervertebral discs.
    e) Tend to involve one joint.

126. A 13-year-old boy with painful mass distal tibia, radiographs shows massive new bone formation has extended into the soft tissue a 'Codman's triangle' on lateral aspect. The likely diagnosis:
    a) Meningioma.
    b) Paget's disease.
    c) Haemangiopericytoma.
    d) Ewing's tumour.
    e) Aneurismal bony cyst.

127. In osteochondritis dissecan's of the knee:
    a) Bilateral in about 85%.
    b) Classic locution is lateral surface of the medial condyle.
    c) Associated with intra articular loose bodies.
    d) MRI is the examination choice.
    e) Joint effusion is almost always present.

128. Solitary bone defect in the skull in a child may be seen in:
    a) Eosinophilic granuloma.
    b) Venous lake.
    c) Chordoma.
    d) Fibrous dysplasia.
    e) Epidermoid.

129. Calcification in ear cartilage (pinna) seen in:
    a) Addison's disease.
    b) Down syndrome.
    c) Amyloidosis.
    d) Diabetes mellitus.
    e) Hypercalcemia.

130. Stress fractures are common in:
    a) The lower tibia.
    b) The lower femur.
    c) The lower fibula.
    d) The neural arch.
    e) The first rib.

131. In Achilles' tendon tears:
    a) The most common ankle tendon injuries.
    b) Diabetes mellitus is predisposing factor.
    c) Associated with gout.

d) Plain radiographs may show obliteration of Kager triangle.
e) Associated with Avulsion fracture of the calcaneus in more than 50%.

132. The following statements are true:
    a) Maffucci's syndrome is a multiple enchordroma with cavernous haemangioma.
    b) Auto-amputation is a feature of ainhum.
    c) Multiple facial osteoma may indicate Gardner's syndrome.
    d) Yaws is a congenital asymmetrical osteoperiostitis.
    e) In sarcoidosis the basic lesion is a caseating granuloma.

133. The best investigation for detection for bone metastasis is:
    a) X-ray alone.
    b) CT scan with plain radiographs.
    c) MRI with CT scans.
    d) X-ray and CT scan.
    e) Bone scan.

134. Complication of prednisone treatment are:
    a) Multifocal avascular necrosis.
    b) Charcot joints.
    c) Bilateral Achilles' tendon ruptures.
    d) Peptic ulcer.
    e) Constipation.

135. In Turner's syndrome:
    a) Increase in the carrying angle of the elbow.
    b) Depressed medial tibial condyle with small beaks on medial corners of methaphyses.
    c) Hypoplasia of atlas.
    d) The pelvic inlet is android.
    e) Long metacarpal bones.

136. Sudeck's atrophy causes:
    a) Painless swelling.
    b) Joint effusion.
    c) Subcortical erosions.
    d) Metaphyseal lucency in young adults.
    e) Hypercalcaemia.

137. Chondroblastoma, the characteristics are:
    a) Margins are not well defined.
    b) Situated in epiphysis.
    c) Diagnosed under 20 years of age.
    d) Painful.
    e) Contains no calcifications.

138. Secondary hypertrophic osteoarthropathy may be seen in:
    a) Carcinoma of bronchus.
    b) Mesothelioma.
    c) Cirrhosis.
    d) Pyelonephritis.
    e) Inflammatory bowel disease.

139. Bony changes on x-ray of patient with polycythemia vera are:
    a) Haemangioma of the brain.
    b) Adrenal pheochromocytoma.
    c) Parathyroid carcinoma.
    d) Mesothelioma.
    e) Myelofibrosis.

140. Myelosclerosis may show:
    a) Periosteal reaction along the femur.
    b) Increased density of the bone only.
    c) Lytic lesions of the bone.
    d) Sideroblastic anaemia.
    e) Lymphadenopathy.

141. Pathological fractures occur in:
    a) Hyperparathyroidism.
    b) Osteitis deformans.
    c) Hemodialysis.
    d) Spina bifida.
    e) Acromegaly.

142. Chondrocalcinosis may be seen in:
    a) Ochronosis.
    b) Fluorosis.
    c) Calcinosis universalis.
    d) Tumoural calcinosis
    e) Hyper parathyroidism.

143. The following are true in dysplasia epiphysialis hemimelica:
    a) Shortening of the affected bone.
    b) Histologically indistinguishable from osteochondroma.
    c) Medial part of the epiphysis usually affected.
    d) The arm is most commonly affected.
    e) When it is multiple usually symmetrical.

144. In crest syndrome:
    a) Swallowing difficulties.
    b) Telangiectasia.
    c) Males are by far more likely to develop limited scleroderma.
    d) Gangrene of fingers and/or toes.
    e) Myocarditis.

145. The following are common in Dressler's syndrome (Post myocardial infarction syndrome):
    a) Plerual effusion.
    b) Paranchymal opacities.
    c) Pericardial effusion.
    d) Leukopenia.
    e) Enlarged cardiac silhouette.

146. Features of myeloma as opposed to metastases are:
    a) Erosion of pedicles.
    b) Generalised osteoporosis.
    c) Elevated serum alkaline phosphatase.
    d) Associated soft tissue mass.
    e) Involvement of nasopharynx.

147. In pigmented Villonudular synovitis of the knee joint:
    a) Knee is the most common site for the disease.
    b) Usually associated with erosion of one side of the joint.
    c) Can diagnosed confidently by plain radiograph.
    d) Lack of particular demineralization is an early sign on plain radiograph.
    e) Change to malignant usually.

148. Pseudofractures (Looser's zone) seen in:
    a) Osteomalacia.
    b) Hyperparathyroidism.
    c) Cleidocranial dysostosis.

d) Osteopetrosis.
e) Spondylolysis.

149. Sacro iliac joint disease can be seen in:
    a) Reiter's syndrome.
    b) Ulcerative colitis.
    c) Regional enteritis.
    d) Mesothelioma.
    e) Paraplegia.

150. Osteitis condensans ilii the following are true:
    a) The sacro iliac joint is usually presented.
    b) Usually seen in multipara over 40 years.
    c) Condition is reversible.
    d) Seen in athletic men.
    e) Can be unilateral.

151. Generalised accelerated skeletal maturation (increased bony age) seen in:
    a) Irradation.
    b) Albright's syndrome.
    c) Pinealoma.
    d) Hyperparathyroidism.
    e) Tuberous sclerosis.

152. Bone within bone appearance seen in:
    a) Iron defeiciency anaemia.
    b) Sickle cell anaemia.
    c) Hypervitaminosis D.
    d) Osteogenisis imperfecta.
    e) Radiation therapy.

153. Localised elongation of bone (overgrowth) seen in:
    a) Hyperemia.
    b) Dysplasia epiphysialis hemimelica (Trevor's disease).
    c) Acromegaly.
    d) Macrodystrophia lipomatosa.
    e) Lymphangioma.

154. Rheumatoid arthritis may present with:
    a) Myopathy.
    b) Encephalitis.
    c) Sudden calf pain.
    d) Large pericardial effusion.
    e) Hypochromic anaemia.

155. The following signs are related to corresponding condition:
    a) Pencil-in-cup sign and psoriatic erosions.
    b) Pencil pointing sign and rheumatoid arthritis.
    c) Pancake kidney (disc kidney) is complete fusion of both kidneys.
    d) Pancake vertebra is vertebra plana.
    e) Putty kidney in hyperthyroidism.

156. In acromioclavicular joint dislocation:
    a) Is synovial joint.
    b) Acromioclavicular ligament is weaker than the coracoclavicular ligaments.
    c) Acromioclavicular joint space is about 1.5 cm.
    d) 50% difference in size between the two shoulders is considered significant.
    e) Separation of the acromioclavicular joint may heal with ossification of the AC ligament.

157. In polyostotic fibrous dysplasia are true:
    a) Commonly causes bone expansion.
    b) Sarcomatous degeneration occurs.
    c) Is usually symmetrical.
    d) There is an elevated serum alkaline phosphatase.
    e) Is associated with delayed puberty.

158. Widening of the lower femoral metaphysis may occur in:
    a) Gaucher's disease.
    b) Pyle's disease.
    c) Thalassemia.
    d) Osteomalacia.
    e) Hemophilia.

159. PVC workers may suffer from:
    a) Sacro-ileitis.
    b) Pulmonary fibrosis.

c) Defects in the middle of the terminal phalangeal shafts.
d) Pneumoconiosis.
e) Mesothelioma.

160. The following are features of sero-positive rheumatoid arthritis:
    a) Myopathy.
    b) Psoriasis.
    c) Encephalitis.
    d) Involvement of metatarso-phalangeal joints without involvement of metacarpo-phalangeal joints.
    e) Pleurisy.

161. Soft tissue calcification occurs in:
    a) Dermatomyositis.
    b) Buerger's disease.
    c) Polyarteritis nodosa.
    d) Paraplegia.
    e) Medullary sponge kidneys.

162. In heel pad thickness:
    a) Is a useful measurement of acromegaly.
    b) Is a useful measurement of hyperthyroidism.
    c) Can be used to assess response to treatment.
    d) Is associated with a plantar spur in more than 50%.
    e) Is measured as the shortest distance from the calcaneum to the skin.

163. In pes cavus (club foot) signs:
    a) Hammer toes.
    b) Claw toes.
    c) Calluses
    d) Hypermobility of the joints.
    e) Compartment syndrome.

164. Following angles are related to:
    a) Cobb angle and the spine in scoliosis.
    b) 'Centre-edge' angle and the hip in femoral acetabular impingement.
    c) Boehler angled and ankle joint in fracture of the calcaneous.
    d) Alpha angle and the hip in femoral acetabular impingement.
    e) Angle of inclination and the spine in scoliosis.

165. Tetany may complicate:
    a) Pyloric stenosis.
    b) Asthma.
    c) Hyperventilation.
    d) Malabsorption.
    e) Ca. rectum.

166. Spontaneous amputation of fingers or phalanges seen in:
    a) Leprosy.
    b) Ainhum.
    c) Streeter's bands.
    d) Asympolia.
    e) Hand-foot-uterus syndrome.

167. The complication of prolonged steroid therapy include:
    a) Nephrocalcinosis.
    b) Avascular necrosis.
    c) Osteomalacia.
    d) Optic atrophy.
    e) Wedge fractures in vertebral bodies.

168. Hypoplastic or short thumb occurs in:
    a) Myostis ossificans progressive (fibrodysplasia).
    b) Thrombocytopenia-Absent Radius (TAR) syndrome.
    c) Triphalangeal thumb.
    d) Apert's syndrome (Acrocephalosyndactyly).
    e) Whistling face syndrome.

169. Abnormal tapering of proximal ends of the metacarpal bones:
    a) Acro-osteolysis.
    b) Epidermolysis bullosa.
    c) Raynaud's disease.
    d) Cornelia de Lange syndrome.
    e) Mucopolysaccharidosis.

170. The following signs or index correspond to following conditions:
    a) Iliac index and mongolism.
    b) Haglund's sign and pulmonary infarction.
    c) Metacarpal sign and Turner's syndrome.
    d) Metacarpal index and arachnodactyly.
    e) Seamoid index and acromegaly.

171. In Milwaukee shoulder syndrome:
    a) Hypermobility of the joint.
    b) Structural damage caused by deposition of calcium hydroxyl apatite crystals.
    c) Superior migration of the humeral head.
    d) Usually bilateral almost symmetrical.
    e) On MRI periarticular marrow edema is a feature.

172. In knee arthrogram:
    a) Can be approached only on the lateral side of the joint.
    b) The site of entry is 2 cm posterior to the patellar midpoint.
    c) It is vital the needle enters horizontally to avoid extra-articular injection.
    d) Patient should walk before images are acquired.
    e) At least 4 images are acquired in each quadrant, and valgus strain should be obtained.

173. MRI shoulder the following are true:
    a) MRI cannot differentiate partial tear from complete tear.
    b) Axial plane is best to demonstrate subscapular tear.
    c) Tears commonly happen just proximal to musculo-tendinous junction.
    d) Contrast arthropathy better seen for adhesive capsilitis.
    e) Intra spinotus is the most common tendon to be torn in the rotator cuff.

174. In monteggia's lesion:
    a) A fracture of the radius.
    b) Dislocation of the wrist.
    c) Intact elbow.
    d) Is a pathological fracture.
    e) Recurrent dislocation of the radial head is recognised complication.

175. In ACL cyst (ACL ganglion cyst):
    a) Usually incidental finding on knee MRI.
    b) Typically high signal T2 MRI.
    c) Typically associated with joint effusion.
    d) Is a sequelae of ACL mucoid degeneration.
    e) Usually multiple and multilocular.

176. In subcapsular femur fracture:
    a) Just distal to the articular margins of the femoral head.
    b) Referred as transcervical fractures.
    c) Garden 1 is a complete fracture without angulation.
    d) The more angulated the fracture is the more likely develop Avascular Necrosis.
    e) In children is commonly due to Perthe's-Legg's-Calve's disease.

177. In patellar dislocations:
    a) More common than patellar subluxation.
    b) Medial dislocation is most common type.
    c) Caused by tracking abnormalities of the extensor mechanism.
    d) Intra-articular dislocation indicate complete quadriceps tendon tear.
    e) Kissing bone contusion pattern indicate medial retinaculum tears.

178. In meniscal tear signs:
    a) Triple PCL.
    b) Two-slice-touch rule.
    c) Double PCL sign.
    d) Absent bow tie sign.
    e) Meniscal flounce.

1. a. True   b. True   c. True   d. True   e. False

Anterior Hip Dislocation
- Hip discoloration accounts for only 5% of all dislocations.
    o Posterior hip dislocations are much more common than anterior dislocations (90% to about 10%).
- Mechanism in anterior dislocation classically occurs when knee strikes dashboard with the thigh abducted, externally rotated with hip flexed.
    o Also falls from a height.
    o Blow to the back while in squatted position.
- Greater force required to dislocate an adult's hip than a child's.

Clinical Findings
- Severe pain, inability to move limb, and numbness.
- Affected limb is sometimes shortened, usually abducted, and externally rotated.
- Signs of vascular or sciatic nerve injury.
    o Pain in hip, buttock, and posterior leg.
    o Loss of sensation in posterior leg and foot.
    o Loss of dorsiflexion (peroneal branch) or plantar flexion (tibial branch).
    o Loss of deep tendon reflexes (DTRs) at the ankle.
    o Local hematoma.

Imaging Findings
- Conventional radiography

- o In anterior dislocations, the head of the femur usually rests inferior and medial to its normal acetabular position, frequently overlying the obturator foramen (inferior type of anterior dislocation).
- o Some anterior dislocations the femoral head may lie superior to the acetabulum (superior type of anterior dislocation).
  - These occur when mechanism is abduction, external rotation, and extension rather than flexion of the leg.
  - The superior type of anterior dislocation may be confused with a posterior dislocation.
- o May be subtle if head in AP plane appears as if it still resides in the acetabulum (superior type of anterior dislocation).
  - These occur when mechanism is abduction, external rotation, and extension rather than flexion of the leg.
  - The superior type of anterior dislocation may be confused with a posterior dislocation.
- o May be subtle if head in AP plane appears as if it still resides in the acetabulum.
- o There may be associated fractures of the anterosuperior aspect of the femoral head (indentation fracture or greater trochanter).
- o Since the anteriorly dislocated head lies farther from the cassette, the anteriorly dislocated head may appear larger than the head on the opposite side, which lies closer to the cassette and is magnified less.

- Computed tomography (CT)
  - o Provides an accurate a means of evaluating not only the dislocation but the associated fractures as well.

2. a. True   b. True   c. False   d. False   e. True

Barton's Fracture
- Intra-articular fracture of the radius with subluxation/dislocation of the wrist.
  - o The lunate maintains its relationship with the fracture fragment.
- May involve the volar aspect of the radius (sometimes called "reverse Barton fracture") or the dorsal aspect.
- Volar type is more common.
- Most common fracture-dislocation of the wrist.

- Dorsal Barton's fracture usually results from fall on an out-streched hand.
- Volar-type is caused by the same mechanism as a Smith fracture.
- Result is deformity at wrist joint.
- Pain, tenderness, swelling and decreased range of motion.
- Conventional radiographs are the study of first choice.
- Fracture is wedge-shaped and extends obliquely on the lateral view into the radiocarpal joint.
- Carpal bones and hand maintain their relationship with the fracture fragment, separating from the remainder of the radius.
- Frequently associated with ulnar styloid fractures.
- CT if further definition is required.
- Colles fracture-extra-articular fracture of the distal radius with dorsal angulation.
- Smith fracture-a fracture of the distal radius with palmar angulation.
   o May have intra-articular component, but dislocation is not a feature as in Barton fracture.
- Galeazzi fracture is fracture of radius with dislocation radio-ulnar joint.
- Bennett's fracture – dislocation the articular surface of the base of first metacarpal is involved and the main portion of the bone is displaced proximally in relation to trapezium.

3.   a. True   b. False   c. True   d. False   e. True

Rickets
- Osteomalacia during enchondral bone growth.
- Age: 4–18 months.
- Clinical findings – irritability, rachitic rosary, bowed legs, delayed dentition/swelling of wrists and ankles.
- Location
   o Metaphyses of long bones subjected to stress are particularly involved: wrists, ankles, and knees.
- Imaging findings
   o Cupping and fraying of metaphysic, poorly mineralized epiphyseal centres with delayed appearance, irregular widened epiphyseal plates (increased osteoid), increase in distance between end of shaft and epiphyseal centre, cortical spurs projecting at right angles of metaphysic, coarse trabeculation (not the ground-glass pattern found in scurvy),

periosteal reaction may be present, deformities common in bowing of long bones and molding of epiphysis.

4. a. True   b. True   c. True   d. False   e. True

Acetabular Protrusio (Protrusio Acetabuli)
- Intrapelvic displacement of the medial acetabular wall.
- Most common cause is osteoarthritis.
- Primary form – Otto pelvis:
  o Usually occurs in young to middle-aged.
  o Bilateral in 1/3 to 2/3 of patients.
  o No underlying causative mechanism is demonstrated.
- Secondary form:
  o Rheumatoid arthritis.
  o Paget disease.
  o Central fracture-dislocation.
  o Osteomalacia.
- May be asymptomatic, or have limitation of motion.
- Joint stiffness.
- Pain.
- Coxa vara and decrease femoral anteversion.
- Joint replacement surgery may be necessary in advance case.

5. a. False   b. False   c. True   d. True   e. True

Erosive (Inflammatory) Osteoarthritis
- Inflammation arthritis that commonly occurs in women over the age of 60.
- It is a form of osteoarthritis with a strong inflammatory component.
- Usually involves hand—swelling, tender.
- Usually begins in DIP joints and progress to PIP joints.
- Typically rheumatoid factor negative.
- Typically bilateral, poly-articular, and relatively symmetrical involvement.
- Central erosion area hallmark resulting in gull-wing appearance.
- Frequent involvement of the carpal-metacarpal joint of the thumb.
- May produce cortical thickening similar to psoriatic arthritis.
- Ankylosis may occur.
- Has been associated with hypothyroidism, autoimmune thyroiditis, hyper parathyroidism, chronic renal disease, scleroderma, Sjögren's syndrome, and calcium pyrophosphate dehydrate arthropathy.

6.   a. False   b. False   c. False   d. True   e. True

Diffuse Idiopathic Skeletal Hyperstosis (DISH)
Ossification of the anterior longitudinal ligament with or without osteophytes is the primary pathology. It is an enthesopathy (there is reaction of the site of tendinous insertions). More common in Caucasian males aged 50–70 years. The ossification is usually quite thick and involves four contagious vertebral bodies. The SI joints are intact differing from ankylosis. The left spine in thoracic area tends to not have ossification of pulsation of the aorta.

Clinical Finding
Back stiffness is worse in the morning.

Large osteophytes can compress or obstruct a number of structures including Bronchus, IVC, oesophagus associated with ossification of the posterior longitudinal ligament also ossification of the vertebral arch ligaments.

Conventional radiography is usually study of choice.

Also involve the pelvis, iliolumbar ligament, iliac crest, ischial tuberosities. There may be ossification of the Achilles' tendon, plantar aponeurosis, triceps tendon, deltoid tuberosities.

7.   a. False   b. False   c. True   d. True   e. False

Osteochondrosis (Osteochondritis) is a disease of one or more epiphyses beginning as a necrosis and followed by healing.

Pathological changes of aseptic necrosis, generally regarded as being due to vascular occlusion.

A traumatic theory is an obvious explanation for some forms, e.g. Osgood-Schlatter's disease, Scheurmann's disease.

Osteochondritis may affect the femoral capital epiphysis (Perthe's-legg's Calve's disease).

In the elbow involve the capitellum in the knee commonly involve the medial femoral condyle.

In the ankle the talus is most usually involved.

Causes of Aseptic Necrosis (some):
1. Perthe's disease.
2. Occlusive Vascular disease (Anteriosclerosis, Thromboembolic disease).
3. Anemia e.g. Sickle Cell disease.
4. Steroid therapy or Cushing's disease.
5. Trauma.
6. Caisson disease.
7. Charcot joints.
8. Collagen disease e.g. Lupus or Poly-arthritis or rheumatoid.
9. Fat embolism (alcoholism).
10. Gaucher's disease.
11. Haemophilia.
12. Gout.
13. Hystocytosis.
14. Drug therapy e.g. Methotrexate – radiation; phenacetin – codeine.
15. Osteomyelitis.
16. Pancreatitis.

Sites of Aseptic Necrosis:
- Femoral Ep. – Perthes.
- Vertebral body – (calve).
- Tibial tuberosity – (Osgood Schlatter).
- Tarsal navicular – (Kohler).
- Second metatarsal mid or 3rd or 4th – (Freigberg).
- Medial tibial condyle – (Blount).
- Vertebral epiphysis – (Scheuermann's disease).
- Calcanela apophysis – (Server).
- Head of humerus – (Hass).

Capitum of humerus – (Panner).

8.   a. True   b. True   c. True   d. False   e. True

Looser lines or Zones or Ostoeoid or called Milkman syndrome is sufficiency stress fractures (incomplete healing due to mineral deficiency).
- Common location, Scapulae (axillary margin) medial femoral neck, shaft of femur ischial rami, ribs.

- Is commonly seen in osteomalacia however other causes such as hypophosphatasia and hyperphosphatasia, osteogenic imperfect tarda, renal osteodystrophy, Paget's disease, stress fracture, fibrous dysplasia including Albright's syndrome.

9. a. False   b. False   c. True   d. True   e. False

Caisson disease (Dysbaric Osteonecrosis) – exposure to a hyperbaric atmosphere whether working in a caisson at tunnel constructing or in deep sea driving may result in decompression sickness and osteonecrosis. It is thought the nitrogen becomes liberated from bone marrow in which it is held in high concentration due to its solubility in fat. Bubbles of liberated nitrogen cause cone infarcts by occluding small blood vessels. Some bony change present related to the joints (Juxtra-articular lesion) dense area, opacities, transradiant subcortical band collapse part of the sequestration. Secondary osteoarthritis commonly.

10. a. True   b. True   c. True   d. False   e. True

Within the sutures of the skull vault small bones may occasionally be seen. They may be multiple in adult and neonate. Either normal or abnormal associated with cleidocranial dysplasia, cretinism, hypothyroidism, osteogenesis imperfecta, Down syndrome, hypophosphatasia progeria, rickets, pyknodysostosis, pachydermoperiostosis.

11. a. True   b. True   c. False   d. True   e. True

The normal thickness of the heel pad is < 2.2 cm. If it thickened bilaterally may indicate obesity, myxedema, normal variant infection of soft tissue e.g. mycetoma, generalized oedema, occupational trauma, acromegaly, drugs e. g. Dilantin therapy.

12. a. True   b. True   c. False   d. False   e. False

Hypertophic Osteoathroscopathy a parallel lamellar new bone formation along diaphysis of the long bones is best seen in the forearms and legs and is rarely marked in the hands. The thoracic cause malignant tumour, bronchogenoic carcinoma, carcinoma of the breast or lung secondaries, e.g., osteogenic sarcoma. It may be benign tumour in the chest, e.g., fibroma, thymoma, haemangioma, or even inflammatory condition such as tuberculosis or lung abscess. The extra thoracic causes include GI tract disease including cirrhosis, chronic active hepatitis, amyloidosis. Also may be associated leukaemia, pancreatic carcinoma.

13. a. True   b. True   c. True   d. True   e. False

Mastocytosis (Urticaria Pigmentosa) systemic disease with mast cell proliferation in skin associated with eosinophilia and lymphocytes. Involve the lamina propria of small bowel lymph glands associated also with most cell leukaemia.

Albright syndrome is fibrous dysplasia skin pigmentation exclusively in females with precocious puberty.

In mycetoma (Madura foot) is a chronic osteomyelitis, the organism is Madura machetes or actiromycosis group of moulds. Diffuse soft tissue swelling are found with skin involvement. Leprosy can cause local destruction of the tufts or digits, pseudocyst or localised bone sclerosis, neuropathic joints, deformity, and disorganisation.

14. a. False   b. True   c. False   d. True   e. False

Bone within the bone appearance seen in several condition including delay of growth e.g. stress, chemotherapy, sickle cell crises. May be seen in normal neonate however ostcopetrosis (marble bone disease) or Paget's disease, or even in hypervitaminosis D, or phosphorous ingestion.

15. a. True   b. True   c. True   d. False   e. False

Nail patella syndrome (familiar osteo-onchodyplasia) is rare autosomal dominant disorder characterised by symmetrical meso-ectodermal anomalies, evident in 2nd + 3rd decades, aplasia/hypoplasia of thumb short 5th metacarpus bone, bilateral posterior iliac horns in 80% is a diagnostic sign. Bilateral spooning or splitting, ridging of fingernails. Fragmented hypoplasia or absence of patella with increase carrying angle with congenital dislocation of radial head, etc.

16. a. False   b. True   c. True   d. True   e. True

Pathological fracture occurs in diseased bones as result of weakness or atrophy, e.g., any causes of osteopenia such as generalised osteoporosis, osteomalacia and rickets, Sudeck's atrophy, and others.

17. a. True   b. True   c. True   d. False   e. False

Volar plate fracture forms floor of PIP joint and separates the joint space from the flexor tendons:
- Volar plate is ligamentous at its origin on to the proximal phalanx.
- Cartilaginous in its insertion onto the middle phalanx.

Hyperextension injury.

Involves PIP joints of fingers.

Primarily a ligamentous injury that can result in fracture.

Injury to the PIP joint is relatively common in athletics, especially sports involving handling, 'jammed finger'.

If force of injury is great enough, dorsal dislocation can occur. Rupture of the volar plate may occur with longitudinal splitting of the collateral ligament structures:
- Allows for complete dorsal displacement of middle phalanx.
- Simple dislocations easily reduced by player coach, or trainer on the field.
- Following reduction, most dorsal dislocations are stable.

Fractures of the base of middle phalanx also occur in association with dorsal dislocations if fracture involves more than 40–50% of articular surface:
- Collateral ligament support is lost
- Combined with coexistent volar plate disruption – represents major loss of joint stability, these injuries are often unstable, existing persistent subluxation of the middle phalanx.

Imaging Findings
- Small fragments of bone is avulsed from palmar (volar) aspect of base of middle phalanx.

18. a. False   b. False   c. False   d. False   e. True

Pachydermoperiostosis (Osteodermopathial) Primary Hypertrophic Osteoarthropathy – Autosomal dominant young male much more than female large thick fold skin of the face and scalp.

May be associated with acroosteolysis. Thick cortex without narrowing of medulla, clubbing fingers, enlarged paranasal sinuses. Irregular periosteal proliferation of phalanges and distal long bones should be differentiated from thyroid acropachy and secondary osteoarthropathy.

19. a. True   b. True   c. False   d. True   e. True

Ostoid osteoma is a benign bone tumour commonly presents between 10 and 38 years, Male > Female. With localised intermittent bone pain of several weeks duration especially at night and typically relieved by Aspirin. Commonly affected the proximal end of femur but any bone may be affected. Bone scanning can be performed increase uptake of the nidus (which occurs centrally).

In osteoblastoma is a benign bony lesion in young adult. The lesion causes pain that differ from ostoid osteoma not occurring characteristically at night and not specifically relieved by Aspirin.

In Brodie's abscess, the lesion is usually found in the cancellous tissue near the end of a long bone. Patient may be symptomatic.

Caries sicca means dry root is cystic bony benign lesion of the head of humerus resemble osteoclastoma.

20. a. True   b. True   c. True   d. False   e. True

Hyperparathyroidism is an excessive production of parathyroid glands (par hormone). Causes a metabolic disturbance characterised by an elevated plasma calcium level. Serum alkaline phosphatase is raised only when bone changes occur. A familial incidence has been described in some cases. It may form part of either type (MEN I and II) of multiple endocrine neoplasia. The main parthyroid lesion adenoma 80%, hyperplasia 15%, and carcinoma 5%.

Types:
1. Primary hyperparathyroidism due to tumour of the gland.
2. Secondary hyperparathyroidism due to hyperplasia of all the glands occurs in response to persistent hypocalcemia of any cause.

3. Tertiary hyperparathyroidism is secondary hyperparathyroidism that develop an autonomous parathyroid adenoma. It may follow osteomalacia or renal failure.

21. a. True   b. False   c. False   d. False   e. False

Caffey's Disease (Infantile Cortical Hyperostosis)
Self-limiting proliferative bony disease of infancy.

Unknown etiology, age < 6 months.

Sudden, hard extremely tender soft issue swelling over bone, irritable, fever, elevated ESR, increase alkaline phosphates, leukocytosis, anaemia. Affects the mandible, clavicles, ulna and other bones. Massive periosteal new-bone formation. Affect the diaphysis of tubular bones, sparing the epiphysis.

22. a. True   b. True   c. True   d. False   e. False

Psoriatic Arthritis
Uncommon disease involving synovium + ligamentous attachments with propensity for sarcoilitis/spondylitis.

Classified as seronegative spondyloarthropathy:
- Positive HLA-B27 in 80%.
- Negative rheumatoid factor.

Psoriatic arthritis resembling rheumatoid arthritis (38%).

Concomitant rheumatoid + psoriatic arthritis (31%).

Widely variable distribution + asymmetry with involvement of lower + upper extremities. Distinctive pattern terminal interphalangeal joints. Unilateral polyarticular asymmetricaldistribution, marginal erosison, no or very minimal Juxtra articular osteoporosis. Destruction of distal interphageal joints, 'pencil-in-cup' deformity (erosion with ill-defined margins plus adjacent proliferation of periosteal new bone).

Rheumatoid arthritis (bilaterally symmetric well defined erosions ± juxta articular osteoporosis).

23. a. False   b. False   c. True   d. False   e. False

a. Giant cell tumour – this lesion is locally malignant an area for osteolytic destruction is found being especially common in the ends of the long bones. Can be cured by excision or curettage, occurs in mature skeleton after epiphysis and presented in 3rd or 4th decade. The sacrum and pelvis are involved occasionally.
b. Aneurysmal bone cyst – presented commonly in 2nd or 3rd decade of life. Prognosis is benign. Can be found every part of the skeleton, rarely involve the vertebral body.
c. Osteoid osteoma, any bone may be affected commonly diaphysis of long bones especially when the spine is affected. The tumour is almost always found in the neural arch and not in the vertebral body.
d. Chondroblastoma arises in the epiphysis of the long bones.
e. Fibrocortical defect or called metaphyseal fibrous defect are metaphyseal in location.

24. a. True   b. True   c. False   d. True   e. True

Generalised increase in bone density in children – the causes of widespread Osteosclerosis in children are many including physiologic Osteosclerosis of newborn. Erythroblastosis fetalis, Gaucher's disease, infantile cortical hyperostosis (Caffey's disease), transplacental infections, e.g., syphilis osteoporosis, pyknodytosis (is combined osteopetrosis and cleidocranial dystosis). Lymphoma and sickle cell anaemia also seen in congenital cyanotic heart disease can be seen in idiopathic hypercalcemia (William's syndrome).

25. a. True   b. True   c. True   d. False   e. False

Osteosclerosis is either localised or generalised.

Physiological in newborn or congenital cyanotic heart disease or unknown, e.g., idiopathic hypercalcemia (William's syndrome).

Also in fluorosis, sickle cell anaemia, osteopetrosis, pyknostosis, fibrous hyperplasia, mastocytosis, lymphoma, osteoblastic secondaries (brest, prostate), Paget's disease, multiple myeloma (rare).

Renal osteodystrophy, tuberous, sclerosis, osteomalacia, healed rickets, hypervitaminosis D, hyperphosphatasis, hyperthyroidism, Engelmann's disease, Caffey's disease, Erythroblastosis fetalis, and many more.

26. a. True   b. True   c. True   d. True   e. False

Periosteal reaction is elevation of the periosteum in different form or either localised or generalised, may be symmetrical. Many layers described onion layers in Ewing's tumour. Sunray speculation may be seen in meningioma, angioma, osteogenic sarcoma, erythroblastic anaemia. The causes are many physiological in premature baby. Congenital in tuberous sclerosis traumatic including battered baby syndrome infection in acute osteomyelitis or in chronic, e.g., Brodie's abscess, varicose ulcer. Hypovitaminosis and hypervitaminosis, rickets, scurvy, hypervitaminosis A.

Endocrine – thyroid acropachy.

Vascular – haemophilia, leukaemia, Hodgkin's disease, collagen disease, e.g., Polyarteritis nodosa, neoplasm, benign meningioma, malignant osteogenic sarcoma, and others, e.g., Still's disease, Caffey's, and histocytosis.

Carcinoma of the bronchus is by far the most common cause of hypertrophic osteoarthropathy.

27. a. True   b. False   c. False   d. True   e. True

Multiple myelomatosis is disease of middle age over 40 years, male more than female. Persistence bony pain or a pathological fracture is usually the first complaints. The serum albumin remains constant so that the albumin-globulin ratio is reversed. Diffuse osteoporosis also can cause suspicion of the disease in elderly patients. Areas of osteolytic lesion usually rounded or oval with poor or well-defined margins may develop. The involvement of the pedicles is possible but commonly seen in metastasis. The classical site of metastasis in the mandible in the mandible is the angle but any part can be involved, myeloma is likely to involve the jaw in the late stages. Myeloma causes vertebral destruction and collapse. It may also extend laterally produce a paravertebral soft tissue mass.

28. a. True   b. True   c. True   d. False   e. True

Hemophilia – due to deficiency of factor VII. This hereditary disease primarily affects males, the gene being carried by females, who exhibit no features of bleeding disorder.

Bleeding into the joints spaces is characteristic, the knee being the joint predominantly subject to traumatic stress and strains, is affected almost invariably frequently bilateral.

The intercondylar notch becomes wide and deep. Other joints also affected hip and elbow. A large soft tissue mass in the soft tissue may void the adjacent bones (haemophiliac pseudotumour).

29. a. False   b. False   c. False   d. True   e. False

Multiple Osteosclerosis bone lesions seen in many conditions including multiple infarct, or bone islands callus (e.g., healed rib fracture), osteoblastic metastasis, chronic healed osteomyelitis, Paget's disease, Olliers's disease, lymphoma, multiple myeloma, tuberous sclerosis, Gardner's syndrome (multiple osteoma).

In plasmacytoma, the bone lesion is solitary in Brown tumour.

In hyperparathyroidism in osteolytic lesion so as in osteoblastoma.

30. a. True   b. True   c. True   d. True   e. False

31. a. True   b. True   c. True   d. True   e. False

32. a. True   b. True   c. False   d. True   e. True

33. a. True   b. False   c. True   d. True   e. False

34. a. True   b. True   c. True   d. False   e. False

35. a. True   b. True   c. False   d. True   e. True

36. a. True   b. True   c. True   d. True   e. False

37. a. False   b. False   c. True   d. True   e. True

38. a. False   b. True   c. False   d. True   e. True

39. a. True   b. False   c. True   d. True   e. False

40. a. True   b. False   c. True   d. False   e. True

41.	a. False	b. True	c. False	d. True	e. True
42.	a. True	b. True	c. True	d. False	e. True
43.	a. False	b. False	c. True	d. True	e. True
44.	a. False	b. True	c. True	d. False	e. False
45.	a. True	b. True	c. False	d. True	e. True
46.	a. True	b. True	c. False	d. True	e. True
47.	a. True	b. True	c. False	d. True	e. True
48.	a. True	b. True	c. False	d. True	e. True
49.	a. True	b. True	c. True	d. False	e. False
50.	a. True	b. False	c. True	d. True	e. False
51.	a. False	b. False	c. False	d. False	e. True
52.	a. True	b. True	c. True	d. True	e. False
53.	a. True	b. True	c. False	d. True	e. False
54.	a. True	b. True	c. True	d. True	e. False
55.	a. True	b. False	c. True	d. True	e. True
56.	a. True	b. True	c. True	d. True	e. False
57.	a. False	b. True	c. False	d. True	e. True
58.	a. True	b. False	c. True	d. True	e. True
59.	a. True	b. True	c. True	d. False	e. True
60.	a. True	b. True	c. True	d. False	e. False
61.	a. True	b. True	c. True	d. False	e. False

62.	a. True	b. False	c. True	d. False	e. True
63.	a. True	b. True	c. True	d. False	e. True
64.	a. True	b. True	c. True	d. False	e. True
65.	a. True	b. True	c. True	d. True	e. False
66.	a. False	b. True	c. False	d. True	e. True
67.	a. True	b. True	c. True	d. False	e. True
68.	a. False	b. True	c. True	d. False	e. True
69.	a. True	b. True	c. False	d. False	e. True
70.	a. False	b. True	c. True	d. False	e. True
71.	a. True	b. True	c. False	d. True	e. True
72.	a. False	b. False	c. False	d. False	e. True

Osteochondrmatosis (Synovial chondromatosis) – mild pain, swelling, and limitation of movement are usual presenting complaints. Cartilaginous masses develop in the suberous layer of the synovium. In the earliest cases an intra-articular effusion may be the only abnormality.

73.	a. True	b. True	c. True	d. False	e. True
74.	a. True	b. True	c. True	d. True	e. False
75.	a. True	b. True	c. True	d. False	e. True
76.	a. False	b. True	c. True	d. True	e. False
77.	a. True	b. True	c. True	d. True	e. False
78.	a. True	b. True	c. True	d. True	e. False
79.	a. True	b. True	c. False	d. True	e. True

Gout – deposition of sodium urate monohydrate crystals in synovial membranes, articular cartilage, ligaments, and bursae leading to destruction of cartilage.

Age of onset is usually greater than 40 years; males much more often than females.
- Idiopathic Gout – M:F = 20:1; overproduction of uric acid; abnormality of renal urate excretion.
- Secondary Gout – rarely cause for radiographically apparent disease; myeloproliferative disorders, e.g., polycythemia vera, leukaemia, lymphoma, multiple myeloma; bloody dyscrasias; myxedema; hyperparathyroidism; chronic renal failure glycogen storage disease; myocardial infarction; lead poisoning.
- Joints: hands + feet (1st MTP joint most commonly affected = podagra), elbow, wrist. Carpometacarpal compartment especially common on knee, shoulder, hip, sacroiliac joint (15% unilateral).
- Ear pinna > bones tendon, bursa.

Radiologic features usually not seen until 6–12 years after initial attack.

Soft Tissue Findings
- Calcific deposits in gouty tophi in 50% (only calcium urate crystals are opaque).
- Eccentric juxtra-articular lobulated soft tissue masses (hand, foot, ankle, elbow, knee).
- Bilateral olecranon buritis.
- Aural calcification

Joint findings
- Preservation of joint space initially.
- Absence of particular demineralization.
- Erosion of joint margins with sclerosis.
- Cartilage destruction late in course of disease.
- Periarticular swelling (in acute monarticular gout).
- Chrondrocalcinosis (menisci, articular cartilage of knee) resulting in secondary osteoarthritis.

Bone Findings
- 'Punched-out' lytic bone lesion ± sclerosis of margin.
- 'Mouse/rat bite' from erosion of long-standing soft tissue tophus.
- 'Overhanging margin' (40%).

- Ischemic necrosis of femoral/humeral heads.
- Bone infarction.

Coexisting Disorders
- Psoriasis.
- Glycogen storage disease Type I.
- Hypo and hyperparathyroidism.
- Down syndrome.
- Lesch-Nylan syndrome (mental retardation, self-mutilation of lips + fingertips).

80. a. False   b. True   c. False   d. True   e. True

Pigmented Villonodular Synovitis
Regarded generally as a benign neoplasm. Adolescents and young adults are affected. Complaining of chronic monarticular pain and swelling around a major joint (knee or hip). The synovial thickening para articular erosions with clearly defined sclerotic margin both sides of the joints are affected. There is preservation of the articular surfaces and the joint space until late stage.

81. a. False   b. True   c. False   d. True   e. True

Osteogenesis Imperfecta
- Hereditary, non-sex linked disorder leading to increased fragility of the bones.
- Hearing loss occurs in half type I individuals.
- Fracture and bruise easily.

Imaging Findings
- Multiple fractures, Wormian bones, beaded ribs, platyspondyly.
- In mild type, there may be thinning of the long bones with thin cortices.
- In more severe, cystic metaphyses, popcorn appearance of the growth cartilages, thin bones, deformities of the long bones due to multiple fractures, rib fractures, and vertebral fractures.

82. a. False   b. False   c. True   d. True   e. True

Sudeck's atrophy is a rare complication of traumatic lesions of the extremities, particularly severe in disuse osteoporosis.

Confined to the bony structures distal to the point of injury. May follow relatively trvial trauma. Present with swelling of soft tissue, smooth severe pain, and immobility.

Symptoms resolve spontaneously in 4 to 8 months with restoration of normal radiological appearance.

83. a. True   b. True   c. True   d. True   e. False

Multiple radiolucent metaphyseal bands may be solitary and may seen in systemic illness or stress in infancy or in utero. Also seen in transplacental infection, e.g., brucellosis, osteogenesis imperfecta, Osteopetrosis, scurvy, Cushing's syndrome.

Hypervitaminosis D is also a recognised cause.

84. a. False   b. False   c. False   d. False   e. True

Progeria (Hutchinson-Gilford Progeria Syndrome)
Premature aging. Typically live to their mid-teen and early twenties. They die from complications, myocardial infarction, stroke, or neoplasm (sarcoma, thyroid carcinoma).

Characterised by generalised soft tissue atrophy, slender long bones, coxa valga, lympoplastic, faciel bone, bilateral cataract, severe osteoporosis, hyperpigmentation. Heart valve classifications with cardiac enlargement, diabetes, hypogonadism.

85. a. True   b. True   c. True   d. False   e. True

Sjogreen Syndrome
- Autoimmune multisystem disorder characterised by inflammation plus destruction of exocrine glands leading to dryness of mucous.
- Affecting the salivary, lacrimal glands mucosa, submucosa of pharynx, tracheobronchial tree, reticuloendothelial system, joints, much common in female.
- Associated with connective tissue disease – rheumatoid arthritis 55%, systemic lupus erythematosis 2%, progressive systemic sclerosis 0.5%, psoriatic arthritis, primary biliary cirrhosis, lymphoproliferative disorders, xeropthalmia (atrophy of salivary gland, parotid gland) is the most common symptom, xeropthalmia

(dryness of eyes), xerorhinia (dryness of nose) and Broncheictasis, rheumatoid factor (positive in up to 95%).

86. a. False   b. True   c. True   d. True   e. True

   A. Lipohaemarthrosis is a term to a condition of fracture bone the release of fat from the marrow cavity and bleeding into a nearby tissue space.
   B. The fat floats on the blood and if a film of the injured area is taken with horizontal ray, a characteristic horizontal level is demonstrated due to the fat-blood interface.
   C. The presence of any posterior fat pad regardless of size and displacement is pathological.
   D. Due to over breathing, due to acidosis, so as in severe asthmatic attack.

87. a. True   b. True   c. False   d. True   e. True

Transverse lines or zones of increased density in the metaphysis may be normally seen in the neonate or systemic severe illness or stress in infancy as well as transplacental infection.

Also in pathological signs of many illnesses, e.g., steroid in high dose, healing scurvy or rickets, treated leukaemia.

Heavy metal or chronic absorption, e.g., bismuth, arsenic, phosphorus, fluoride, mercury lithium, and radium. And Methotrexate therapy or parathyroid therapy. Oestrogen in high dose or heavy metal during pregnancy. Seen also in hypervitaminosis D and hypothyroidism, parathyroid therapy, idiopathic hypercalcemia.

88. a. False   b. False   c. False   d. False   e. True

Triplane Fracture – the fracture involves the frontal, lateral, and transverse planes. It extends sagittally through the epiphyseal plate and coronally through the distal tibial metaphysis. Occurs in older children/young adolescents in 18 months just prior to epiphyseal plate closure. Mechanism of injury is forced external rotation. They may be classified by the number of fragments into two-part, three-part, and four-part triplane fractures.

Localised pain, swelling, inability to fully bear weight, ankle deformity.
- Conventional radiography is the study of first choice.
- CT is helpful in optimally demonstrating all of the fracture fragments and their relationships.
- Two-part fracture appears on lateral view as if it were a Salter-Harris IV fracture.
- Three-part fracture appears as if it were a Salter-Harris III fracture on AP view and as if it were a Salter-Harris II fracture on lateral view.

Differential Diagnosis
Tillaux fracture – Salter-Harris III fracture involving the distal tibial epiphysis however, displaced fractures, and most three-part triplane fractures require operative reduction and internal fixation.

Epiphyseal arrest and angular deformity are uncommon.

89. a. False   b. False   c. False   d. False   e. True

Pelvic Rib or Digit
- Rare congenital anomaly.
- Bone develops in soft tissue.
- Can arise from any of the pelvic bones; also anterior abdominal wall, most commonly arises from ilium.
- Unilateral.
- Usually asymptomatic; discovered incidentally.

Imaging Findings
- Digit or rib has cortex and medulla
- 'Finger' is typically segmented with peudo-articulations.

Fong's disease (onychoosteodysplasia) – iliac horns is a rare Autosomal dominant disorder characterised by abnormal pigmentation of iris renal dysfunction, bilateral posterior iliac horns in 80% occasionally capped by an epiphysis; short 5th metacarpal; scoliosis, genu valgum.

90. a. True   b. True   c. False   d. False   e. True

Epidermal Inclusion Cyst
- Associated with trauma, especially penetrating trauma.

- Usually in bones that are superficially located such as fingers, foot, and calvarium.
- Implantation of epithelium that form cysts leading to bone erosion.
- Sublingual crush-type injuries have been associated with inclusion cysts as has prior surgery.
- May develop within weeks or years of fingertip injury.
- Pain at the site of lesion.
- Mass.
- Frequently seen in terminal phalanx.
- Solitary, lytic lesion.
- May be expansile.
- May have a thin sclerotic border.

Differential Diagnosis
- Echondroma, metastasis (rare), glomus tumour.

91. a. False   b. False   c. True   d. True   e. False

Sternomanubrial Dislocation
- Usually occurs with high energy impact.
- Can occur with lower impactforces if there is a pre-existing arthropathy, e.g., rheumatoid arthritis or sever kyphosis
- Fracture through manubrium without dislocation can occur.
- Suspected clinically, instability, deformity, severe pain over sternomanubrial junction.
- Lateral chest radiographs or CT scan confirms diagnosis.
- On CT, other potentially life-threatening injuries to aorta, great vessels, trachea, and oesophagus may be seen.
- Upper thoracic spine and rib fractures share the hyperflexion mechanism injuries.
- Stable, uncomplicated injuries are treated with closed reduction.
- Unstable injuries and those with an associated mediastinal injury may require open reduction.

92. a. False   b. False   c. False   d. False   e. True

Necrotizing Fasciitis
- A rapidly progressive, infection of fascia that leads to subsequent necrosis of the subcutaneous tissue, muscles are frequently spared.
- It may be caused by several organisms of groups of organisms including Clostridial infections (gas gangrene).

- Frequency may be increasing because of immunocompromised patients.
- Organisms spread from subcutaneous tissue along both superficial and deep fascial planes.
- Intense pain, sometimes out of proportion to the physical findings, and tenderness over involved area.
- After a few days, nerve necrosis may produce anesthesia in the area, a clue to the presence of necrotizing fasciitis.
- Edema, skin vesicular eruptions, and crepitus.
- Lymphagitis and lymphadenitis are infrequent.
- Plain films are insensitive to the presence of gas in the soft tissues so that a negative conventional radiograph should not rule out the diagnosis.
- Non-enhanced CT is the study of choice and may show thickening of fascial planes and gas in the subcutaneous tissue.
- MRI can be sensitive in determining the presence of necrosis and need for surgical debridement, combined with clinical evaluation.
- Ultrasound may reveal subcutaneous collections of air and fluid not otherwise seen.
- Necrotizing fasciitis associated with diabetic.
- May be idiopathic, as in scrotal or penile necrotizing fasciitis (Fournier Gangrene).
- Hyperbaric oxygen treatment may be helpful.

93. a. False   b. False   c. False   d. True   e. False

Giant Bone Island
- Bone islands (enostoses) are areas of mature compact bone in cancellous bone in the medullary cavity. Usually oriented with its long axis parallel to the cortex.
- Most common pelvis, proximal femurs, and ribs. Dense round or ovoid. Greater than 2 cm in size.
- Speculated, feathered, or brush-like margin. Thickening of trabecula.
- Radionuclide bone scan usually shows no increased uptake.
- MR – loss of signal on all sequences.
- It may be confused:
  - Osteoblastic metastatic disease.
  - Osteosarcoma.

94. a. False   b. True   c. True   d. True   e. False

Melerheostosis (Leri's Disease, Flowing Periosteal Hyperostosis)
- Melorheostosis is sclerosing bone disorders of unknown causes:
  - Produces thickening of the endosteum and periosteum.
  - Peak age of presentation is 5–20 years.
  - May be monostotic common in lower extremities.
- Adult present with pain, joint stiffness, deformity that may progress over time.
- Children may present with leg length discrepancies, joint contractures, resembling osteoma.
- Candle-wax appearance (classic), myositis ossificans, osteopathia striata.
- Usually in the diaphysis, that resemble 'candle-wax-dripping'.
- Cortical hyperostosis with an undulating appearance usually affecting one side of a bone.
- Soft tissue lesions that may calcify adjacent to involve bone.
- May grow to compress nerves.
- Bone scan is markedly positive.

Differential Diagnosis
- Osteopathia – longitudinal dense striations.
- Osteopoikilosis – punctuate, rounded bone islands surrounding joints.
- Osteosarcoma – bone destruction.

Associated soft tissue lesions and cutaneous lesions: vascular malformations, neurofibromatosis, tuberous sclerosis, haemangioma, muscle contractures, scoliosis.

95. a. False   b. True   c. True   d. True   e. False

Fibrous Dysplasia
- Most common 3–15 years is replacement of medullary bone by fibrous tissue. Shepherd's crook deformity of femur.
- Most commonly involved bone are pelvis, femora.
- In widespread disease, the skull and jaw are almost always involved. Plain x-ray, endosteal scalloping, cortical thinning, ground-glass appearance, may have matrix calcification.
- Prone to fracture.
- Growth of lesions usually stops when epiphyses close.
- Albright's syndrome – Polyostotic, sexual precocity, skin pigmentation, almost always in a female.

96. a. True   b. True   c. True   d. True   e. False

Ankylosing spondylitis is chronic inflammatory disease unknown etiology primarily affecting spine.

Mostly Caucasian male 15–35 years, presented with insidious onset of low back pain and stiffness.

HLA-B 27 positive immune than 90% sacroiliac joint involvement bilaterally bamboo spine, squaring vertebra, apophyseal, and costovertebral ankylosis is marginal syndesmophyte formation. Vertebra planna does not occur in ankylosing spondylitis, is seen in osteochondritis or eosinophilic granuloma, etc.

97. a. True   b. False   c. True   d. True   e. True

Rheumatoid Arthritis is generalised condition which affects the collagen of the tissue in many parts of the body in addition to the joints.

Incidence between 40 and 60 years.

Women > Men.

The radiological signs may classified:
- a. Changes in the soft tissue, e.g., symmetrical fusiform swelling around the joints, while eccentric in gout arthritis.
- b. Osteoporosis – juxtra-articular.
- c. Erosion.
- d. Changes in the joint space:
    1. Early stage – widen
    2. Later stage – narrowed

98. a. False   b. True   c. True   d. True   e. True

Fingertips Calcifications
- Can be anywhere in the hands some calcifications about the fingertips.
- Occur in scleroderma, dermatosis, calcinosis universalis, epidermolysis bullosa, lupus erythematosis, Rathmund's syndrome, Raynaud's disease.

99. a. False   b. False   c. False   d. True   e. False

Vascular calcification associated with phleboliths seen in normal, varicose veins, haemangioma, Maffucci's syndrome, post radiation.

Vascular calcification can occur in many other causes however phleboliths not present such as frostbite, gout, hypervitaminosis D, Buerger's disease, aneurysm, atherosclerosis hyperparathyroidism, homocystinuria, idiopathic hypercalcemia, immobilisation syndrome, milk-alkalin syndrome, Sarcoidosis, Takayasu's arteritis, and pseudoxanthoma elasticum.

100. a. False   b. True   c. False   d. False   e. True

Anterior Shoulder Dislocation
- Young individuals
- External rotation and abduction.
- 40% recurrent.
- May be associated with fracture of greater tuberosity 15%, Bankart lesion – fracture of the anterior glenoid rim, and Hill-Sachs defect (impacted fracture of posterolateral surface of humeral head due to impaction of humeral head against anterior rim of glenoid during dislocation).

101. a. True   b. True   c. True   d. False   e. True

Carpal Tunnel Syndrome
- Entrapment syndrome caused by chronic pressure on the median nerve within the carpal tunnel
- Causes pressure effect by Nasser cysts however flexor tendon tendinitis or tenosynovitis.
- Presented with finger paresthesias, clumsiness, weakness, nocturnal hand discomfort.
- Diagnosed best by MRI pseudoneuroma of the median nerve (swelling median nerve proximal to carpal tunnel) swelling of the median nerve within the tunnel. Increase signal intensity of the nerve on T2W1.
- Volar bowing of flexor retinaculum swelling of tendon sheath due to tenosynovitis.

102. a. True   b. True   c. True   d. False   e. False

Achondroplasia
- Autosomal dominant or sporadic mutation disorder of abnormal enchondral bone ossification
- Most common form of short-limbed dwarfism (less than 3rd percentile in standing height)

In Achondroplasia, the extremity involvement is rhizomelic (i.e. proximal) so that the humerus and femur are more involved than the radius and tibia.

Clinical Findings
- Delayed motor development
- Recurrent otitis media
- Normal intelligence
- Short stature
- Lower extremity radiculopathy

Imaging Findings
- Can be detected before birth by the use of prenatal ultrasound
- After birth, conventional radiography is the study of first choice
- Skull
    o Frontal bossing
    o Enlarged calvarium and mandible
    o Hypoplasia of the midface
- Hands and feet
    o Short phalanges
    o Fingers of equal length (trident hand)
- Spine
    o Narrowing of the interpediculate distance
    o Thickening and shortening of the pedicles
        ▪ Narrowed AP diameter
    o Decreased height of vertebral bodies
        ▪ Anterior wedging may produce a 'bullet' shape
- Pelvis
    o Squared iliac wings
    o Narrow sacroiliac notches (champagne glass appearance)
    o Reduced acetabular angle
- Long bones
    o Bones are short (rhizomelic) and wide
    o Genu varum
    o Widening of the metaphyses
    o Posterior bowing of the distal humerus

Differential Diagnosis
- Diastrophic Dysplasia
- Spondyloepiphyseal Dysplasia

103. a. True   b. True   c. True   d. False   e. False

Non-union Fracture
- Delayed union is the term applied when a fracture has not healed within the period of time that would be considered adequate for bone healing for that particular sites.
- Non-union is the term applied to a fracture that will not unite without additional intervention.

Associations
- Open or compound fracture.
- Degree of comminution.
- Less soft tissue covers fracture.
- High energy fractures (automobile and motorcycles accidents).
- Cigarette smoking places patient at higher risk.
- Use of nonsteroidal anti-inflammatory medications may inhibit bone healing.

Types
A. Hypertrophic non-unions
   - Exuberant callus formation.
   - Because of their vascularity, they have excellent healing potential.
   - Result from adequate immobilisation of the fracture.
B. Atrophic (Oligotrophic) non-unions
   - Absence of callus and bone ends that may be tapered and osteopenic or sclerotic.
   - Because of their lack of vascularity, they have poor healing potential.
   - A subcategory of this type may be freely movable and form a pseudoarthrosis.
C. Normotrophic non-unions
   - Share characteristics of both of the above.

Imaging findings
- Conventional radiographs are the study of first choice.
  - Is established non-union, the ends of the fracture fragments are sclerotic and typically smooth.

- Bones are joined by fibrous tissue.
- CT may be helpful in establishing presence of bony bridging.
- MRI is most sensitive for osteomyelitis.

104. a. True   b. True   c. True   d. False   e. False

Coxa vara is displacement of the head of femur in relation to the metaphysis almost always in a posteromedial direction.

The femoral head situated low in the acetabulum, secondary deformity of the acetabulum result from malposition of the femoral head.

The infantile caoxa vara called cervical coxa vara. The adolescent coxa vara called epiphysiolosis or slipped epiphysis.

The causes of coxa vara are many including Perthe's-Legg's disease, Paget's disease, rheumatoid arthritis, rickets, osteomalacia, fibrous dysplasia, osteoporosis, congenital hypoplasia of femur, and others.

105. a. True   b. True   c. False   d. False   e. False

Pigmented Villonodular Synovitis is reagarded generally as a benign neoplasm.

Adolescents and young adults are affected usually complaining of chronic monarticular pain and swelling around a major joint, usually the knee or hip.

Radiologically, the synovial thickening is clearly evident, especially with soft tissue exposures. Para-articular erosions with clearly defined sclerotic margins. Both sides of the joint are affected and presentation of the articular surfaces and the joint space until the late stage of the disease.

Lack of periarticular demineralization.

106. a. True   b. True   c. False   d. False   e. True

Diaphyseal aclasia is hereditary and familiar condition is presence of cancellous exoctosis containing a cartilaginous cap and by a failure of bone modeling resulting in expansion of bone ends.

The epiphysis never affected.

The common sites are bones around the knee however any bone can be affected.

Pressure symptoms on bones, vessels, and nerves may be found, about 5% of cases change to malignant.

107. a. True   b. True   c. True   d. True   e. False

108. a. True   b True   c. True   d. False   e. False

109. a. True   b. False   c. False   d. True   e. True

Tarsal Coalition / Talar Break

General Considerations
- Rare (1% incidence).
- Fusion of two or more tarsal bones in the hindfoot (talus and calcaneous) or midfoot (cuboid, navicular, and cuneiforms).
- Most common coalitions (90% of total) are calcaneous and navicular (calcaneonavicular) and calcaneous and talus (talonavicular).
- Fusion may be congenital or acquired.
  o Congenital form is familial – Autosomal dominant with near complete penetrance, bilateral 50% of time, and more common in males than females.
  o Acquired form may be due to trauma, infection, arthritis surgery.

Types
- Complete coalition – bony (synostosis).
- Incomplete coalition – cartilaginous (synchondrosis); fibrous (syndesmosis).

Clinical Findings
- Most are asymptomatic.
- When symptomatic, symptoms begin in 2nd decade of life, made worse by physical activity.
- Restricted range of motion.
- Muscles spasms.

Imaging Findings
- Conventional radiography of the foot is the study of first choice.
- Calcaneonavicular fusions should all be evident on a 45° internal oblique view – bridge is usually from anterolateral aspect of calcaneous to dorsolateral aspect of navicular.
- With fibrous and cartilaginous coalition, the joints may be narrowed, sclerotic, and irregular.
- Talocalcaneal coalition may be more difficult to see:
    o Most common involves junction between the middle facet of the talus and the sustentaculum talus.
    o Talar beak presumably occurs because of limitation of emotion in subtalar joint—at insertion of talonavicular ligament, periosteal reaction develops and beak not present in all patients with talocalcaneal coalition.
- Pes planus deformity is common.
- Hypoplasia of the sustentaculum tali may occur.
- MRI is most sensitive to fibrous and cartilaginous fusion.

110. a. True   b. False   c. True   d. True   e. True

Ewing Sarcoma

General Considerations
- Second most common malignant bone tumour in children (after osteosarcoma).
- Accounts for approximately one-third of all primary bone tumours.
- More common in males than females – more common in Caucasians.
- Occurs between the ages of 5–30 years. Highest frequency between 5 and 15 years. Rare over age 30.
- Location:
    o Arise in medullary cavity, usually of long bones in the lower extremities.
    o Most commonly occurs in long bones and pelvis – more occur in femur, pelvis, tibia, and humerus.
    o But they can occur virtually any bone.
    o Commonly involves metadiaphysis of long bones.

Clinical Findings
- Most common symptoms are localised pain and swelling.

- Additional symptoms may include fever, weight loss, anaemia, leukocytosis, and elevated erythrocyte sedimentation rate.

Imaging Findings
- Most lesions are visible on conventional radiographs. However, their degree of spread is better evaluated with MRI.
- Common manifestations on conventional radiography include:
    o Poorly marginated, lytic, destructive lesion – Permeative (small holes) or moth-eaten (mottled) appearance. Rarely, they can be sclerotic.
    o Soft tissue mass or infiltration is common – soft tissue mass may occur without destruction of cortex. Soft tissue mass may produce saucerization (scalloped depression in cortex).
    o Periosteal reaction is common – lamellated – onion-skinning due to successive layers of periosteal development. Sunburst or speculated – hair-on-end appearance when new bone is laid down perpendicular to cortex along Sharpey's fibers. Codman's triangle – formed between elevated periosteum with central destruction of cortex.
    o Osteosclerosis may be present secondary to reactive bone formation.
- Other, less common, manifestations – thickened cortex, expansion of bone, and pathologic fractures.
- Radioisotope bone scan – increased uptake in areas of bone destruction. Whole body bone scans are used to detect metastatic lesions. Metastases may be present in up to 30% of cases at time of diagnosis.
- CT – to evaluate bone destruction and extra-osseous involvement.
- MRI – method of choice for tumour staging. Assesses soft tissue involvement – low signal intensity on T1W1. Heterogeneous gadolinium enhancement. High signal intensity on T2W1. Evaluates response to chemotherapy and radiation treatment.

Differential Diagnosis
1. Neuroblastoma
2. Leukaemia, reticulum cell sarcoma, multiple myeloma
3. Osteomyelitis
4. Eosinophilic granuloma
5. Osteosarcoma
6. Lymphoma

111. a. True   b. True   c. True   d. False   e. True

112. a. False   b. True   c. False   d. False   e. False

Cleidocranial Dysostosis / Cleidocranial Dysplasia
- Rare, congenital hereditary resulting in delayed or failed ossification of midline structures.
    o Especially membranous bones, but enchondral bones are also affected, therefore, skull and clavicles are mostly affected.
- Autosomal dominant with strong familial tendencies.
    o Males and females have same chance of being affected.
    o Gene for this disorder has been found on chromosome 6.
    o May also occur as sporadic mutation.
- Major changes are in the skull, clavicles, and pelvis.
- Large head; disproportionate small facial bones; narrow chest; sagging shoulders; may be dwarfism of defensive dentition; and no mental retardation.

Imaging Findings
- Skull
    o Wormian bones – intersutural bones, especially seen in the lambdoid and posterior sagittal sutures.
    o Large head.
    o Thinness and under ossification of calvarium in the early infancy.
    o Widened fontanelles and sutures with delayed closure
    o Persistent metopic suture – midline suture in frontal bone.
    o Brachycephaly and prominent bossing.
    o Large mandible – non-union of mandibular symphysis.
    o High marrow plate; may be cleft.
    o Hypoplastic paranasal sinuses, including mastoids.
    o Delayed or defective definition – abnormally retained primary teeth.
    o In adulthood, petrous bones may be sclerotic.
- Chest
    o Hypoplasia or absence of clavicles – clavicle normally forms from this ossification centres: sterna, middle and distal; one or more segments in any combination may be absent - usually of lateral portion and R > L; clavicles completely absent in 10%.

- o Thorax may be narrowed and/ or bell-shaped – small scapulae.
- o Supernumerary ribs.
- o Incompletely ossified sternum.
- Spine
    - o Hemivertebrae, spondylosis (frequent).
    - o Exaggerated kyphosis or lordosis.
    - o 'Bone-within-a-bone'.
- Pelvis
    - o Delayed ossification of bones forming symphysis pubis – produces widened symphysis.
    - o Hypoplastic iliac bones.
    - o Poorly formed sacrum.
- Extremities
    - o Accessory epiphyses in hands and feet were common.
    - o Coxa vara from deformed or absent femoral necks is common – broad femoral head and short femoral neck.
    - o Radius short or rarely, absent.
    - o Elongated second metacarpals.
    - o Pseudoepiphyses of metacarpal bases.
    - o Short hypoplastic distal phalanges of hands.
    - o Pointed terminal tufts.
    - o Coned epiphyses.

Differential Diagnosis
- Widening of symphysis can be seen with bladder exstrophy.
- Calvarial and clavicular changes in pyknodysostosis can be identical to cleidocranial dysostosis but bones are sclerotic in pyknodysostosis.
- Short or absent radius may be seen with Holt-Oram syndrome or TAR syndrome.
- Absence or erosion of the distal clavicle can be seen with rheumatoid arthritis, hyperparathyroidism, and scleroderma.
- Bone-within-a-bone can be seen with osteoporosis, Paget's disease, and with Thorotrast administration.
- Wormian bones can be seen with hypothyroidism, Down syndrome, cretinism, pyknodysostosis, and osteogenesis imperfecta, but are most often a normal variant.

113. a. True   b. True   c. False   d. True   e. True

Complex Regional Pain Syndrome (Sudeck's Atrophy / Reflex Sympathetic Dystrophy)
- Most causes occurs secondary to fractures, sprains, and minor soft tissue injury includes head injury, stroke, myocardial infarction, cast/splint immobilisation.
- When involves nerve injury is called causalgia.
- Edema is most common sign continuing pain, allodynia, or hyperalgesia.

114. a. True   b. True   c. True   d. False   e. True

115. a. True   b. True   c. False   d. True   e. False

116. a. True   b. True   c. True   d. False   e. True

117. a. True   b. True   c. True   d. True   e. False

118. a. False   b. False   c. False   d. True   e. True

Fibrous dysplasia is a benign tumour-like congenital process, manifested as a localised defect in osteoblastic with progressive replacement of normal bone with immature woven bone.

119. a. True   b. False   c. False   d. True   e. False

Unicameral Bone Cyst / Simple Bone Cyst / Solitary Bone Cyst
- Common (3–5% of primary bone tumours).
- Benign.
- Solitary lesion.
- Most common in proximal humorous and femur – also iliac bone and calcaneous, especially over age 20.
- Most common between 4 and 10 years old – Male:Female – 3:1.
- Filled with clear yellowish fluid – may contain giant cells and hemosiderin.
- Asymptomatic.
- If fractured, then pain and limited range of motion.

Imaging Findings
- Conventional radiography is the study of choice.
- Most common in proximal humerus (in patients under 20) and femur in skeletally immature male.

- Solitary, lytic metaphyseal lesion adjacent to, but not crossing, the epiphysesal plate – migrates towards diaphysis during growth of child.
- Well define margins with narrow transition zone.
- May be slightly expansile.
- Long axis of lesion is parallel to long axis of bone.
- May have thin sclerotic margin.
- Endosteal scalloping and erosion.
- Fallen Fragment Sign represents a fragment of the bone that falls into the cyst and then into a dependent position. Although uncommon, it is pathological for a cyst because it indicates the fluid nature of the interior of this lytic lesion.
- On CT, they may be shown to contain air-fluid levels.
- On MRI, they will have low signal intensity on T1 and high on T2 – lesions which have fractures will have a heterogeneous signal on T1 and T2 because of the hemosiderin. Their periphery may enhance with Gadolinium.
- Photopenic on bone scan.

Differential Diagnosis
- Fibrous dysplasia – ground-glass; more irregularly shaped.
- Eosinophilic granuloma – look for other lesions, bevelled-edge, vertebra plana.
- Chondoblastoma – extends into epiphysis
- Brown tumour – is locally destructive areas of intense osteoclastic activity. May occur anywhere in the skeleton and may expand the bone, this seen in hyperparathyroidism.
- Aneurismal bone cyst – more expansile.
- Enchondroma – smaller bones, internal calcifications.

Treatment
- Curettage and bone grafting, nailing, injection of bone marrow or cryotherapy to prevent pathologic fracture.
- Methylprednisolone injections have been used to promote healing.

Complications
- Pathologic fractures in 50–65%.
- Growth arrest in affected limb.

Prognosis
- Usually undergo spontaneous regression.

120. a. False   b. False   c. True   d. False   e. True

Calcium Hydroxyapatite Depositon Disease (HADD) calcium phosphate crystals are deposited in the form of calcitic tendinitis. The shoulder is the most common site. Maybe bilateral presented with pain, limitation of motion. Plain radiograph shows homogeneous sharply defined, well-circumscribed amorphous collections of calcium density without trabeculation, near the joint usually. MRI finding low signal focus on all sequences calcification can also be in elderly women (Milwaukee shoulder).

121. a. True   b. True   c. False   d. True   e. True

Also fatty liver, gallstones bile duct carcinoma. Amyloitosis, urolithiasis oxalate/uric acid, acid stones, and erythema nodosium.

122. a. True   b. True   c. True   d. False   e. False

123. a. True   b. True   c. True   d. False   e. False

Hair loss also occur in alopecia arenta, anaemia, burns, syphilis, hormone changes, tumour of ovary, and adrenal gland. Birth control pills, beta blockers, calcium channel blockers, antidepressants drug.

124. a. False   b. True   c. True   d. True   e. True

Also seen in association with acromegaly, diabetes mellitus, it may be familial.

125. a. True   b. True   c. False   d. True   e. False

126. a. False   b. False   c. False   d. True   e. False

Codman's triangle is extension of periosteal reaction indicative of farther spread of tumour along medullary cavity. Can occur in metastases, haemangioma, TB, and tropical ulcer. Also in mycetoma. Also in older people in Paget's, meningioma.

127. a. False   b. True   c. True   d. True   e. False

128. a. True   b. True   c. False   d. True   e. True

Single or multiple also seen in cranium bifidum, meningocele, encephalocele, dermal sinus, lacunar skull, neurofibromatosis, parietal foramen, hydatid, osteomyelitis, tuberculosis, haemangioma. Tumours primary, e.g., Ewing's or metastasis, e.g., lymphoma. It may be traumatic, e.g., Burr hole, depressed fracture, leptomeningeal cyst, etc.

129. a. True   b. False c. False   d. True   e. True

Also seen in gout, acromegaly collagen disease, frostbite, trauma, sarcoidosis, polychondritis hypopituitarism, hypoparathyroidism, hypercoticism, dwarfism, etc.

130. a. True b. False c. True d. True e. True

Stress fracture (Fatigue fracture) the constant or repeated stress from which they result is very often some form of athletic or occupational activity. Radiolograph may show a hairline translucency of a crack fracture usually running transversely across the bone. Commonly affected the metatarsal necks (March fracture). Also the middle or lower part of the tibial shaft (common in male ballet dancers). Lower fibular fracture of this type is associated with long-distance running and that of the upper shaft with jumpers from height as in the repeated training for parachute jumping. Lower ribs stress fracture in mid axillary line from chronic cough. The first ribs from carrying a heavy pack. The calcaneous and clavicle are also a sites for fatigue fracture.

131. a. True   b. True   c. True   d. True   e. False

Also associated with ochronosis, hyperparathyroidism repeated including system, lupus erythematosis.

132. a. True   b. True   c. True   d. True   e. False

133. a. False   b. False c. False d. False e. True

Radioisotope bone scan is the preferred method for the detection of bone metastasis. Technetium-99m is the commonly used radioisotope. It accumulates in reactive new bone that is formed in the metastases resulting in a hot spot in the scan. The amount of accumulation depends on the level of the blood flow in some cases cold spots noted due to absence of bone formation within the lesion. The results from a bony scan are not specific as the tracer can accumulate in other areas with increase bony formation such as site of old fracture or infection.

134. a. True   b. True   c. True   d. True   e. False

135. a. True   b. True   c. True   d. True   e. False

136. a. False b. False c. True   d. True   e. True

137. a. False b. True   c. True   d. True   e. False

138. a. True   b. True   c. True   d. False   e. True

Secondary Hypertrophic Osteoarthropathy (HPOA) – radiological feature of parallel Lamellar new bone formation along the diaphyses of the long bones is best seen in the forearms and legs and is rarely marked in the hands.

The lesion is usually bilateral symmetric causing swelling and extreme pain of the affected limbs.

The primary condition that is familiar and affect mainly males.

139. a. True   b. True   c. True   d. False   e. True

140. a. True   b. True   c. False   d. True   e. True

141. a. True   b. True   c. True   d. True   e. False

142. a. True   b. True   c. False   d. False   e. True

143. a. True   b. False c. True   d. False   e. True

144. a. True   b. True   c. False   d. True   e. True

Limited Scleroderma (Crest syndrome) is a variant of progressive systemic sclerosis (PSS) and stands for:
   C - Calcinosis
   R - Reynaud's phenomenon
   E - Esophageal dysmotility
   S - Sclerodactyly
   T - Telargiectasia

145. a. True   b. True   c. True   d. False   e. False

146. a. True   b. True   c. False   d. False   e. False

147. a. True   b. True   c. True   d. True   e. False

148. a. True   b. True   c. False   d. False   e. True

149. a. True   b. True   c. True   d. False   e. True

150. a. True   b. True   c. True   d. False   e. True

151. a. False   b. True   c. True   d. False   e. True

152. a. False   b. True   c. True   d. False   e. False

153. a. True   b. True   c. False   d. True   e. True

154. a. True   b. True   c. True   d. True   e. False

155. a. True   b. True   c. True   d. True   e. False

Pencil pointing sign is commonly at the end of the clavicles. Putty kidney in autonephrectomy due to renal tuberculosis.

156. a. True   b. True   c. False   d. True   e. True

Distance between AC joint is usually < 5 mm.

Coracoacrominal ligament is denser, thicker, and stronger than AC ligament.

Stress views of injured and uninjured shoulders help in diagnosis of type 1 injury (sprain).

157. a. True   b. True   c. False   d. False   e. False

158. a. True   b. True   c. True   d. False   e. True

159. a. True   b. False   c. True   d. False   e. True

160. a. True   b. False   c. False   d. True   e. True

161. a. True   b. True   c. True   d. True   False

Also seen in aneurysm, arteriosclerosis, nephritic syndrome, diabetes, burn, frostbite, gout, hypervitaminosis D, hyperparathyroidism, Werner's syndrome, Hypoparathyroidism, etc.

162. a. True   b. False   c. True   d. False   e. False

163. a. True   b. True   c. True   d. False   e. True

164. a. True   b. True   c. True   d. True   e. False

Angle of inclination and the hip joint for coxa vara deformity and coxa valga, increased stress on hip.

Carrying angle of the elbow for gunstock deformity supracondylar fracture.

Lateral talocalcaneal angle for varus deformity of foot and club foot.

165. a. True   b. False   c. True   d. True   e. False

166. a. True   b. True   c. True   d. True   e. False

Ainhum is an unknown cause in African fissure constriction across the soft tissue that leads to fracture separation and tapered ends and auto amputation.

Asympolian congenital indifference to pain streeter's bands syndrome is congenital amniotic bands, constriction of soft tissue causing oedema and osteopenia distally, and auto amputation.

167. a. True   b. True   c. True   d. False   e. True

168. a. True   b. True   c. False   d. False   e. False

Hypoplastic thumb also seen in phocomesis, e.g., thalidomide poisoning. Seen also in Holt-Oram syndrome, Basal cell nevus syndrome (Gorlin), hand-foot-uterus syndrome, Trisomy 18 syndrome.

Thumb may be enlarged in triphalangeal and angioma, neurofibromatosis. The thumb may be ectopic in whistling face syndrome also called flexed thumb over laps palm. The thumb may be wide in Apert's syndrome, Carpenter's syndrome, and ostopalatodigital syndrome.

169. a. False   b. False   c. False   d. True   e. True

The distal ends tapering occurs in all causes of Acro-osteolysis, diabetes mellitus, epidermolysis bullosa, leprosy, hyperparathyroidism, Raynaud's disease, scleroderma, thermal injury, and others.

170. a. True   b. False   c. True   d. True   e. True

Seasamoid index defined as the diameter of the medial seasamoid of the first metacarpophalangeal joint multiplied by the greater perpendicular measurement (the radiograph performed at a 36-inch focus-film distance).

Acromegaly is present when this value exceeds 40 in men and 33 in women.

Iliac index obtained by adding the iliac angle to the acetabular angle. If the iliac index is under 60, mongolism is very probable.

Metacarpal sign in Turner's syndrome normally the line extending tangentially from the distal ends of the 4th and 5th metacarpals should pass distally to the head of third metacarpal. If the 4th metacarpal bone is short, such a line will either just touch or pass through the head of the third metacarpal.

Metacarpal index in Marfan's syndrome (arachnodactyly).

Estimation of the metacarpal index will aid the diagnosis in doubtful cases. By measuring the lengths of the second, third, fourth, and fifth metacarpals and dividing by their breadths taken at the exact mid-points. The resulting figures from each of the metacarpals are added together and divided by four.

In normal adult subjects the metacarpal index varies from 5.4 to 7.9.

In arachnodactyly the range varies from 8.4 to 10.4.

Haglund's sign represent prominence of posterior, superior Calcaneal tuberosity mostly in females from pressure by shoes.

171. a. False   b. True   c. True   d. False   e. True

Capsular. Tendinous, ligamentous, and bursal calcification are common in patients with calcium hydroxy apatite crystals.

The disease can progress to tenderness, swelling, and restricted motion and joint disorganisation with deformity.

172. a. False   b. True   c. False   d. True   e. True

173. a. False   b. True   c. True   d. True   e. False

174. a. False   b. False   c. False   d. False   e. True

Monteggia's lesion is a complex injury that is composed of a fracture of the ulnar shaft associated with a dislocation of the radial head.

175. a. True   b. True   c. False   d. True   e. False

ACL ganglion cysts arising from the alar folds that cover the infrapatellar fat pad. It make up the vast majority of intra-articular ganglion cyst of the knee. May be asymptomatic, often multilocular centred on distal ACL.

176. a. True   b. True   c. False   d. True   e. False

Classification of intracapsular hip fractures:
- Garden I – incomplete or impacted fracture.
- Garden II – complete fracture without displacement.
- Garden III – complete fracture with varus angulation.
- Garden IV – complete fracture with total displacement.

177. a. False   b. False   c. True   d. True   e. True

178. a. False   b. True   c. True   d. True   e. True

www.ingramcontent.com/pod-product-compliance
Lightning Source LLC
Chambersburg PA
CBHW020725180526
45163CB00001B/109